Contents

U222 $18⁹⁵

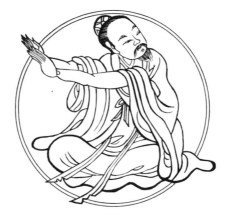

Chinese
Healing Arts
Internal Kung-Fu

Edited by William R. Berk

Originally translated by John Dudgeon, M.D.

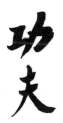

ISBN: 0-86568-083-3

A large portion of this book appeared originally under the title
The Beverages of the Chinese; Kung-Fu or Tauist Medical Gymnastics
translated and annotated by John Dudgeon, M.D., and
published by the Tientsin Press in Tientsin, China in 1895. The
woodcuts also appeared in this volume.

DISCLAIMER

Please not that the publisher of this instructional book is
NOT RESPONSIBLE in any manner whatsoever for any injury
which may occur by reading and/or following the instructions
herein.

It is essential that before following any of the activities,
physical or otherwise, herein described, the reader or readers
should first consult his or her physician for advice on whether
or not the reader or readers should embark on the physical
activity described herein. Since the physical activities described
herein may be too sophisticated in nature, it is *esential that a
physician be consulted.*

Unique Publications
4201 Vanowen Place
Burbank, CA 91505

功夫 Foreword

This book is drawn largely from Chinese classical literature translated in the late nineteenth century by Dr. John Dudgeon, a British physician who lived in China for nearly twenty years. During that time he was a professor of Western Anatomy and Physiology at the Imperial College in Beijing. His avocation was documenting Chinese culture, philosophy and history; Dudgeon wrote nearly thirty essays on all aspects of Chinese life. The healing arts held his greatest interest, and Dr. Dudgeon liked to compare Chinese medical practices to Western theories and procedures.

Although Dudgeon was not a practitioner of martial arts, he did an excellent job of translating this material. Oral traditions and a specific vocabulary, handed down from generation to generation, lie outside the mainstream of daily vocabulary. Translation of old texts in any language is difficult, but it is especially difficult in a language as highly pictured and esoteric as Chinese. Unfortunately, because Dudgeon was not a practitioner of these arts, he failed to understand certain exercises, in particular Taoist sexual techniques. Afraid of offending his reading public (primarily Victorian British), and not understanding the true value of the exercises, he did not translate portions of the older manuscripts.

The material translated by John Dudgeon nearly one hundred years ago is seldom taught today, even in the Far East, except by a few masters. Many of these Kung-Fu methods are well-guarded secrets, and often these techniques are handed down very, very selectively. A variety of procedures are covered in this volume: meditation, concentration, respiratory exercises, static and dynamic posturing, gonadal control techniques, herbal prescriptions to maintain health and cure illness, kneading, percussion with instruments to inure the body with strength and energy, and acupressure. Certain exercises have never been published before in English, including the muscle and tendon modifying techniques, and the marrow washing techniques of Bodhidharma which are partially included in this book.

Healing and martial arts go hand-in-hand in China. The five elements of Chinese medicine are earth, water, metal, fire and wood. In harmony these elements produce sound health; out of harmony they produce various diseases and disorders. Some martial arts intend to harmonize the five elements, and the practice of these arts will bring optimum health. Meditative techniques produce not only mental clarity and spiritual fulfillment, but also increase the good health of the practitioner. Certain meditative techniques eliminate blocked energy and benefit circulation.

It is not uncommon at high levels of the martial arts for the teacher to talk more about healing arts than fighting arts, more about meditative arts than military arts, and more about ethics and morals than about "kicking ass." By learning breath control and internal exercises, we are trying to attain total health: mental, spiritual and physical. If you have a totally integrated being, you become a fearsome warrior, if the need arises. Hopefully, the need will not arise, but the fighting spirit of the warrior will be with you in your daily life, and will help you accomplish daily tasks.

Fine old Chinese texts on martial arts and internal training were always intended by their authors to show the existence of special knowledge, and never the step-by-step procedure for attaining it. Books should be a guide to help locate the correct lineage, school and sifu. It is best to learn from a respected teacher. Some techniques require diligent practice and close supervision to affect dramatic changes in the constitution. Given casually in book form, some exercises could cause injury, illness, or no results at all.

The practice of Kung-Fu means hard work, patience and dedication, over a long period of time. Through hard work and dedication the student goes through stages to a metamorphosis. The student's whole body system, mental set, and sometimes spiritual connections with the universe get organized and reorganized in different patterns, which may put stresses and demands on the nervous system and the whole body. If the teacher is systematic, the student will be spared some of the miseries of training, such as soreness and the contusions caused by accidental blows. If the teacher is very knowledgeable, the student will be spared the mental anguish that may be caused by meditation. Becoming a martial arts expert is not easy; it is a very difficult job for the teacher, and extremely difficult for the novice practitioner.

Sometimes the novice expects to learn so-called secrets so that he can magically control any situation. Unfortunately, too much material has been written which says, "In a few easy lessons, you too can become a master." The study of martial arts is similar to the study of a musical instrument. There is lesson progression, starting from the basic understanding of music, through the study of musical scales, harmony, and simple songs to more difficult compositions. The study of Kung-Fu must also begin with the most basic theory and follow the instruction of the teacher.

The teacher tries to motivate the student to practice as much as possible so that he can benefit from the lessons. The more practice, of course, the easier it is for the teacher to help the student on his path. Traditionally, martial arts disciplines are taught slowly, and the student must develop the patience illustrated by the teaching methods of his master. Students must be checked very carefully to make certain lessons are not taught prematurely. In the fighting arts, for example, you don't match a novice with an experienced fighter. The novice could get hurt or "gun shy," and their future progress might be limited. Basic sparring techniques and knowledge are increased slowly, so that eventually, when the student faces an opponent, hopefully, the student can be on equal ground. These methods encourage the student.

My teachers expected tremendous amounts of dedication from their students, but at the same time, they didn't want their students to make martial arts their whole life. Students were expected to be responsible to their families and work, show interest in other art forms, learn proper etiquette, etc. They were trying to create in their students well-rounded personality.

I discovered that the longer I studied with my teachers, the so-called secrets, the more esoteric aspects of the arts were taught to me. I came to realize I had to have proper understanding, proper mental set, and that my physical body needed to be capable of enduring the hardships of the new lessons. Usually, when I was ready to learn a new topic, it was presented to me. Sometimes I would ask in advance. My teacher would respond, "In time I will, if you dedicate yourself to what I've already shown you."

You insult your teacher by undervaluing his lesson, if you do not practice it to perfection. If you just practice a little and want the teacher to show you something new, you are indicating you don't appreciate his instruction. You are only looking into the future, when he might show you something you will appreciate. Instead of only looking to the future, the novice-practitioner should totally immerse himself in the techniques from the very beginning. It is a real joy to practice beginning-level techniques in this manner, and this type of practice will better prepare the student for the future and more rigorous practice.

It is very important for a martial artist, or anyone looking for exercises to promote good health and possible longevity, to practice seriously all the exercises you learn. It is not theory that will make you more proficient as a martial artist, and it is not knowledge that will make you healthier. Only dedicated practice will accomplish these goals. Practice is the solution, not knowledge; but it is the knowledge which enables you to be on the proper course. And it is the grace of having a qualified teacher that enables you to learn the right knowledge at the right time.

I will be glad at any time to pass knowledge on to those who are truly interested in finding a legitimate master, as often these teachers do not seek publicity. In my own case, I travelled for over seven years and interviewed hundreds of teachers until I found the few that could help me genuinely understand and attain the goals I had always hoped were possible.

ACKNOWLEDGMENTS

I would like to thank my friends and associates for their help and guidance in this project. I can never repay my teachers, who are truly masters, for their kind tutelage. At most, I can show them that their lessons were appreciated, by my continued practice and increased ability to perform the exercises properly. Joan Iten Sutherland, who updated the romanization, checked for historical accuracy, translated the anatomical charts, and did the calligraphy and research for the herb index, helped make this information accessible to the modern student. We owe a debt of gratitude to the masters of the past who developed these brilliant exercises. Finally, I'd like to thank my wife who travelled with me on this journey, who has also learned, practiced and appreciated the martial arts, and is in her own right very competent. For without a fellow traveler along this path, there would indeed have been lonesome times.

CAUTION

Experimenting with any exercise without the proper guidance can be extremely dangerous. Improperly performed, the exercises may produce no results and may even cause injury or illness. I will gladly furnish the names and locations of schools for anyone who is interested in becoming a student. Please write to William R. Berk, P.O. Box 1220, Palm Springs, California 92263.

Chinese herbal medicine is not to be taken lightly. Some of the prescriptions may cause harm, if taken by the wrong person or at the wrong time. Consult with a qualified Chinese doctor on all matters pertaining to your health.

功夫 Introduction

The first mention in Chinese history of a system of movements proper to maintain health and cure disease refers back to prehistoric times, during the reign of the Great Yü, when the country was inundated, the atmosphere was nearly always wet and unhealthy, and disease overflowed, so to speak, the earth. The Emperor ordered his subjects to take military exercise each day. The movements which they were thus obliged to make contributed not a little to the cure of those who were languishing, and to maintaining the health of those who were well.

Emperor Yü instituted the dances named *Ta Wu* 大 舞 , the Great Dances. It was believed that Human life depends upon the union of heaven and earth. The subtle material circulates in the body; if the body is not kept in movement, the humours do not flow, matter collects, and disease originates from such obstruction. The great philosophers explained the cause of maladies in a similar way. But what is especially remarkable in the Chinese tradition is that moisture and stagnant water are considered the source of endemic and epidemic maladies, and that an efficient means of preventing them consists of the regular exercise of the body, or of the circling dances. These movements tend to produce a centrifugal result, very suitable to restoring the functions of the skin and giving tone and vigour to the whole being. These dances form part of the institutions of China.

We read also in the *Shu Ching* (Classic of History) that Emperor Yü ordered the dances to be executed with shields and banners. These two sorts of dances were the first sanctioned in the *Li Chi* (Book of Rites), a work on civil and religious ceremonies. Great importance was attached to regular bodily exercises. As in Greece, learning to sing and dance well constituted a good education.

The founder of the Shang dynasty (c. 1766 B.C.) had engraved in the bathtubs: "Renew thyself each day completely; make it anew, still anew, and always anew" 苟 日 新 日 日 新 又 日 新 .

From the earliest times, the six liberal arts (music, arithmetic, writing, religious and civil ceremonies with their dances, fencing, and charioteering) were taught in public institutions. We read in the life of Confucius that he applied himself to the perfection of all these exercises. Regular and rhythmic movements were engaged in to maintain health and to combat certain diseases.

Even before the period of movement for the cure of disease was the period of healing by the virtues of plants, according to Chinese tradition. Although the legendary Fu-hsi had begun to cure maladies in this way, the art is particularly ascribed to the equally legendary Shen-nung. He distinguished a great many plants and determined their different properties; the first *Great Herbal* is ascribed to him.

Up to the present day, the people exercise in order to give themselves bodily strength and as much suppleness as possible—as in, for example, the exercises of the bow and arrow; throwing and catching a heavy stone with a hole cut in as a handle, heavy bags of gravel, or a bar with two heavy stones at the ends; the various feats of jugglery, etc. This taste for bodily exercise is one of the fundamental elements in that which is still considered the base of all progress and moral development: the improvement of one's self.

The term *Kung-fu* 工 夫 means "work-man," the man who works with art; to exercise oneself bodily; the art of the exercise of the body applied to the prevention or treatment of disease; the particular postures in which certain Taoists hold themselves. The expression *Kung-fu* 功 夫 is also used, meaning "work done". The term *Kung-fu*, "labour" or "work," is identical in characters and meaning with the word *Congou*, applied in the South to a certain kind of tea. In China it is applied medically to the same subjects as are expressed by the German *Heil Gymnastik*, or Curative Gymnastics, and the French *Kinesiologie*, or Science of Movement. Among the movements which are embraced by this method are massage, friction, pressure, percussion, vibration, and many other passive movements, the application of which, when made with intelligence, produces essential hygienic and curative results. These different movements have been in use in China since the most ancient times. They are employed to dissipate the rigidity of the muscles occasioned by fatigue, spasmodic contraction, rheumatic pains, the effects of dislocations, fractures, and edema.

These practices have today passed into the habits of the people, and those who are in charge of them are usually the village healers who frequent the streets, advertising their presence by striking a kind of tuning fork called *huan-tou*. Those who usually practice these movements are the healers who have medicine shops, and the various exercises are generally gone through in the mornings and evenings. There is also a class of masseurs who go to private houses or who undertake to teach the art. Here we certainly have a procedure allied to medical gymnastics, to which the Chinese attribute therapeutic value.

Kung-fu embraces, as already remarked, massage (from the Greek *massein*, "to rub," or Arabic *mass*, "to press softly"), and shampooing (a Hindu word meaning "to knead"), a highly esteemed practice still in vogue in China. Massage consists of such operations as kneading, thumping, chafing, rubbing, pressing, pinching, etc. The masseurs, as a part of their duty, treat their customers to a kneading of the scalp, eyebrows, spine, calves, etc. These operations are practised both for the prevention and cure disease, but also more generally, as in Western countries, for the comfort and sense of bracing which it confers. The various methods of manipulation comprised under the term massage include *effleurage*, *petrissage*, *friction*, and *tapotement*. All these movements are centripetal, and done with the dry hand. The effect produced by such manipulations is the promotion of the flow of lymph—otherwise designated *humours* by the older writers—and blood, and the stimulation of the muscles and the skin reflexes.

Mere rubbing or shampooing is no more massage than a daub of paint is a work of art. It is not only a vicarious way of giving exercise to patients who cannot take it themselves, but it is also a valuable curative agent. Lady Manners, in the *Nineteenth Century*, says, "The Chinese are supposed to have learnt the use of gymnastic exercises from the Indians, and the subject mentioned in the most ancient of their books is called *Cong-fow*, or Science of Living."

The Taoists, the priests of the religion or system of Lao-tzu (c. 500 B.C.), have always been the chief practitioners of this form of medical gymnastics. These Taoists were the early alchemists of the world, and for centuries had been in search of the philosopher's stone. In cinnabar they supposed they had found the *elixir vitae*. Alchemy was pursued in China by these priests of Tao long before it was known in Europe. From approximately 200 B.C. to at least 400 A.D., the transmutation of the base metals into gold and the composition of an elixir of immortality were questions ardently studied by the Taoists. The Arabs, in their early intercourse with China, thus borrowed it and were the means of its diffusion in the West. Kung-fu owes its origin to these same investigators, and it was adopted at a very early period to ward off and cure disease and to strengthen the body and prolong life, for which it has been declared a far-reaching and efficacious system.

It is the object of Kung-fu to make its votaries almost immortal; at least, if immortality is not gained, it is claimed that it tends greatly to lengthen the span of life, to increase the body's power of resistance to disease, to make life happier, and to make the muscles and bones insensible to fatigue and the severest injury, accidents, fire, etc. Also, the benefit the soul derives from such exercises and the merit accruing to the individual are not to be lightly esteemed.

Kung-fu consists of two things, the posture of the body and the manner of respiration. There are three principal postures: standing, sitting, and lying. The priests of Tao enter into the greatest detail about all the attitudes in which they vary and blend the different postures. The different modes, in the three principle positions, of stretching, folding, raising, lowering, bending, extending, abducting, and adducting the arms and legs form a numerous variety of attitudes. The head, the eyes, and the tongue each have their movements and positions. The tongue is charged with performing such operations as balancing, pulsating, rubbing, shooting, etc. in the mouth, in order to excite salivation. The eyes close, open, turn, fix, and wink. The Taoists pretend that when they have gazed at the root of the nose for a long time, first on one side and then on the other, the torrent of thought is suspended, a profound calm envelops the soul, and they are prepared for a doing-nothing inertia which is the beginning of communication with the spirits.

Regarding respiration, there are three modes—one by the mouth, one by the nose, and inspiration by one and expiration by the other.

The constituents of Kung-fu have now been presented. It lies with art to choose and combine them, to change and repeat them according to the malady for which a cure is sought. The morning is the best time for it. After a night's sleep, the blood is in a state of greater repose and the humours are more tranquil, especially if one has been careful to sup lightly. Fat persons should eat nothing at night, and this preparation is absolutely necessary for certain maladies.

In Pére Amiot's *Notice du Cong-Fou* (1779), twenty figures are given to illustrate the text. In each of the postures, the principal thing is to respire a certain number of times in a particular manner, and to proportion the length of the Kung-fu to the malady. The body is either half nude or dressed, and the position is either standing or sitting. There are series of each. In respiration, the mouth must be half full of water or saliva. Various potions, decoctions, and drugs are ordered to be taken before or after Kung-fu; they seem to have been added in the course of time, to facilitate the effects. In a few words, Amiot indicates the different maladies which the postures are said to cure.

The physical and physiological principles of the art are the following.

1. That the mechanism of the human body is hydraulic.
2. That the air, which enters the blood and the lymph through the lungs without cessation, as the balance which tempers and restores their fluidity, can neither be re-established nor subsist of itself.

The consequences of these two principles are:

1. That since the circulation of liquids in the human body has to conquer the two great obstacles of weight and friction, everything which tends to diminish one or the other will aid in re-establishing it when it is altered.
2. As physical activity increases, the flow of body fluids (blood, lymph, etc.) is stimulated.

There are two essential principles of Kung-fu—the posture of the body, and the mode in which respiration is quickened, retarded, and modified.

1. If we look at the circulation of the blood and lymph, and the obstacles which the weight opposes to it, it is evident that the mode in which the body is straight or bent, lying or raised, the feet and hands stretched or bent, raised, lowered or twisted, ought to work a physical change in the hydraulic mechanism which facilitates or impedes it. The horizontal situation, which diminishes the greatest obstacle of weight, is also the most favourable to the circulation. That of being upright, on the contrary, leaving all its resistance to the action of the weight, ought necessarily to render the circulation more difficult. For the same reason, depending on how one holds the arms, the feet, and the head—raised, inclined, or bent—it ought to become more or less easy for the circulation. This is not all; that which retards it in one palce, gives it more force where it does not find any obstacle; and, from that time, it assists the lymph and the blood in overcoming the engorgements which obstruct their passage. One can further add that the more it has been impeded in one place, the more its impetuosity brings it back there with force when the obstacle is removed.

It follows from this that the different postures of Kung-fu, well directed, ought to operate in a salutary disengagement in all the maladies which spring from a retarded, or even interrupted, circulation. Now, how many complaints are there that are not thus caused? One can even ask if, excepting fractures, wounds, etc., which derange the bodily organisation, there are any which do not so originate.

2. It is certain that the heart is the prime mover of the circulation, and the force which it has to produce and conserve is one of the grand marvels of the world. It is further certain that there is a sensible and continual correspondence between the beatings of the heart, which fills and empties itself of blood, and the movements of dilatation and contraction of the lungs, which empty and fill themselves with air by inspiration and expiration. This correspondence is so evident that the beating of the heart increases and diminishes immediately, in proportion to the acceleration or retardation of the respiration. If we inspire more air than we expire, or *vice versa*, its volume ought to diminish or augment the total mass of blood and lymph, and ought to invigorate more or less the blood in the lungs. If one hurries or retards the respiration, one ought to hurry or weaken the beatings of the heart.

The bearing of this on Kung-fu is self-evident. It is obvious that, in accelerating or retarding the respiration, we accelerate or retard the circulation, and by a necessary consequence that of the lymph; and that, in the case of inspiring more air than we expire, we diminish or augment the volume of the air which is therein contained. Now, all this mechanism being assisted by the posture of the body, and by the combined and assorted positions of its members, it is evident that this ought to produce a sensible and immediate effect upon the circulation of the blood and lymph.

The animal forces, locomotive or muscular—*Yang*—and the vegetative forces, secretory or chemical—*Yin*—are harmonized and held in equilibrium by the physical forces, *T'ai-ch'i*; from this state of equilibrium result life and health. These three forces have contrary tendencies; the *Yang* tends to produce and perpetuate itself incessantly, the *Yin* tends to descend to the terrestrial region, and the *T'ai-ch'i* remounts to its origin, the *Tao*, the reason of all visible manifestation. The *Yang* and the *Yin* are so united that they are in a state of reciprocal dependence, and they possess only a certain power of reaction proportioned one to the other, a power dispensed by the *T'ai-ch'i*.

It is to the maintenance of this proportionality—this species of static, physical, chemical, and intellectual equilibrium—that the will, human moral power, and the acts by which this will manifest itself, ought to tend incessantly. Kung-fu has been instituted for this object. It is charged with the maintenance or re-establishment of all parts of the body and its faculties in their condition of unity and primitive harmony among themselves and with the soul, in order that the soul may have at its disposition a powerful and faithful servant for the execution of its will. In other words, and from the *Notice* of Amiot, Kung-fu is "a real exercise of religion, which, in curing the body of its infirmities, frees the soul from the servitude of the senses," and gives to it the power to accomplish its duties upon the earth and to raise itself freely to the perfection and perpetuity of its spiritual nature in the *Tao*, the reason of the grand creative power.

Thus Kung-fu, in its primitive institution, appears as a reminder of the Tree of Life, to which humans of the first days came, after their labours, to shelter their forces and health and to conserve their souls, still pure, a docile instrument of their will. Such are the principles upon which the Chinese theory of Kung-fu reposes, like that of their chemical and pharmaceutical medicine, and also that of their religions, social, and philosophic doctrines; for the Chinese, whatever their studies of people or the institutions which concern them may be, always carry their considerations into all the elements of their nature and constitution. However we may think that the progress of the civilization of the West has not yet arrived at this degree of practical reason, we are certainly astonished to see that, from the first ages of humanity, the priests of *Tao* were in possession of this grand thought of the unity of human nature, and that they had made the application of it to all things, even to hygiene and to therapeutics, by movement organised in its relations with the physical, chemical and psychical laws of the human being.

I am indebted for much of what has now been presented, in illustration of this system, to Pére Amiot, and particularly to M. Dally, who has published a large work on the subject called *Cinesiologie ou Science du Movement* (Paris, 1857), in which he reviews Amiot's *Notice*.

This art is a very ancient practice of medicine, founded on principles originally pure and free of all the superstition with which it is today surrounded. It goes back to a period when Taoist priests formed an official sacerdotal caste, in the time of the legendary Huang-ti (c. 2698 B.C.). The art consists of three essential parts:

1. It comprises divers positions of the body and the art of varying the attitudes; it explains how, during these positions and attitudes, the

act of respiration ought to be carried out, following certain rules for various inspirations and expirations.

2. The method has its own scientific language.

3. It has operated in the cure of disease, and in the alleviation of many infirmities.

The Chinese, to whatever order they belong, make eager recourse to this mode of therapeutics, when all other means of cure have been tried in vain. Thus, Kung-fu has all the characters of an ancient scientific method.

功夫 Physiology of Kung-Fu

The general principles of this art may be briefly and clearly expressed in the following quotation from one of the numerous Chinese works on the subject, and from one of the prefaces written in commendation of the system.

The Chinese acknowledge three principles or forces upon the regular arrangement of which human life depends—the vital spirits *Ching* 精 , or organic forces, produce the animal spirits *Ch'i* 氣 , or forces, and from these two springs a finer sort, free from matter and designed for the intellectual operations, termed *Shen* 神 . The particles of the vital spirits glide over one another as does water; growth and nourishment belong to them. The animal spirits put the internal and external senses into exercise; their particles are smaller than the vital and they move in every sense like particles of air. Since it is not possible to subsist without these forces, care must be taken not to dissipate them by immoderate involvement in sensory pleasures, by violent efforts of the body, or by too great or too constant application of the forces or spirits. In addition, they have two organic principles, which pervade all parts of the body, from the union of which the human being is made and life depends. The one is *yang*, vital heat, light, the male principle; the other is *yin*, radical moisture, darkness in nature, the female principle.

The body is divided into right and left, the pulse on each side governing its own half of the body. The internal parts are divided into the five viscera[1] and six *fu*[2]. There are six which lodge the radical moisture and belong to the female principle, comprising the heart, liver,

[1]Heart, lungs, spleen, liver, and kidneys, related to the female principle.
[2]Organs connected with the outer air: gall bladder, stomach, large and small intestines, bladder, and the three divisions, related to the male principle.

and left kidney, all situated on the left side, and the lungs, spleen, and right kidney [otherwise called the "gate of life," but by other writers this latter expression is more correctly applied to the vagina] on the right. Those which contain the vital heat are on the left—the small intestines, pericardium, gall bladder, and ureters; on the right are the large intestines, stomach, and the three divisions of the trunk [altogether imaginary]. Certain relations are supposed to exist between these—as, for example, between the small intestines and heart, gall bladder and liver, ureters and left kidney, on the left side; or large intestines and lungs, stomach and spleen, three divisions and right kidney, on the right side. These organs contain the vital heat and radical moisture which go from them into all the other portions of the body by means of the spirits and blood. All the various members of the body, the diseases, the materia medica, etc., are arranged according to a well-established and ancient relation between them and the Five Elements, five colours, five tastes, five points of the compass, etc.

Each organ has a road or blood vessel proceeding to it, and as there are twelve Chinese divisions of time [each one comprising two of our hours] in a day, and as the blood and air make a circuit of the entire body in twenty-four hours, the blood remains in each organ two hours. There are twenty-three roads or vessels and, of course, as many pulses, one for each vessel and organ. These pulses are subdivided into male and female according to the dual principle, and this, it is evident, involves three double pulses on each side; thus the theory is elaborated. Still further divisions of the pulse are made, into superficial, deep, and intermediate, according to whether the pressure of the finger is applied lightly, firmly, or intermediately to indicate diseases of a superficial, deep, or intermediate position. Numerous volumes exist in Chinese on the pulse alone, on the skill of which subject the Chinese pride themselves, as it is the pivot upon which their whole system turns.

As an example, take the pulse of the large intestines. It belongs to the male principle and is felt at the "foot" [cubit, the third pulse position at the wrist reckoning from the base of the thumb backwards] on the right arm. (The small intestinal pulse is felt at the same spot on the left arm.) The blood flowing to the large intestines rises at the tips of the thumb and index finger, unites and flows up the back of the arm to the head, then down the face to the lungs, and thence to the intestines; in the larynx it gives off two branches which run upwards to the ear, across to the mouth, and terminate at each side of the nose. Deafness, ringing in the ears, or pain behind the ears and in the arms are owing to the large intestines. The blood resides in this viscus from 5 to 7 o'clock A.M.

At first the yin [earthly vapour] and yang [heavenly air] produced the root of the human being, the kidneys; one of another of the Seven Ch'ing 情 [3] [emotions or passions] injures the original air and so causes disease. Thus the circulating air of the entire body gets blocked up, the blood gets coagulated in heaps, and then disease is produced; therefore in ancient time good people who understood the Great Reason [Tao] sought out clear methods by which to nourish the original air. Kung-fu was discovered in this way, and as the bear carries his neck firmly and the birds use their wings, so must the eyes and ears be directed inwards and the air and blood conducted to the joints to nourish them. Thus what is above will flow below and what is below will flow upwards. As the heavenly elements are themselves strong and fixed, so must we try to bring our bodies into the same condition; as the heavenly bodies are always revolving according to the Divine Law, so must the air in our bodies. The creation of the great heaven must resemble the creation of the little heaven.[4]

In a small work by a native of Soochow named P'an Wei-wei 潘霨偉 , Wei-sheng-i-chiu-cheng, written in the year 1858, the following prefatory remarks on Kung-fu occur:

Why do some people live and others die? Why are some diseases light and others severe? To answer these questions, we must refer to the existence in sufficient or insufficient quantity of the original vital principle. The origin and foundation of the five viscera depend upon the spring from the vital principle.[5] It is here that the yin and yang reside, from where these male and female principles emanate, and whence the breath proceeds in expiration and to which it goes in inspiration. There is no fire nor oven, and yet the body in its furthest parts is kept quite warm; there is no water nor reservoir, and yet the five viscera are kept moist.

Everyone must beware of admitting depraved air—as, for example, heat, cold, and such like—into the five viscera and six fu, the twelve

[3]The Seven Ching are the following: joy injures the heart; anger, the liver; grief, the lungs; doubt, the spleen; fear, the kidneys; anxiety, the gall bladder; and sadness and crying, the spirit of the liver and air of the lungs.
[4][Ed. note: i.e., the microcosm (the human being) should be like the macrocosm (the universe), a basic principle of alchemy throughout the world.]
[5]The Taoists believe that the original source of Being and Life is situated in and comes from a point in the abdomen, called tan-t'ien, one inch below the navel. The Medical Faculty believe it is to be found in the lumbar vertebrae, at a point opposite the kidneys, immediately adjoining the side of the spinal column, opposite the "small heart," or supra-venal capsule. It is also called on this account the ming-men or "gate of life."

arteries and veins, tendons, blood, and flesh; otherwise, if such poison-ous air should gain admittance, disease will be contracted.

The ancients used acupuncture and the moxa[6] as remedies; after-wards they took stones and rubbed themselves in order to cause the blood to flow. They also used friction to the skin and muscles by the hand to cure disease and cause the blood and air to move. They also used a more violent pressing and rubbing method over the affected part. They also had a spirit-drink mode. All these methods were designed to cause motion in the joints—to harmonize the blood and air so as to leave no vacuum and to cause the depraved air to escape and be quickly expelled, because only on its exit will the perfect and wholesome air be revived as before, circulate, and so secure freedom from disease.

When disease is expelled, great care must be taken with the *tan-t'ien*, so that the original fire and water may coalesce and assist each other; the individual's spirit will then wax greater and stronger, and the bad air cannot enter. But one must not on any account wait until disease has attacked the system and is unbearable. It will then be too late. True wisdom is to begin Kung-fu before the approach of the disease, and so prevent it. It is true that the limit of our lives is fixed, but at the same time it is also true that the body can be strengthened by Kung-fu. This is therefore the object of this publication. The author has consulted the work of *Hsu Ming-feng* 徐 鳴 峯 and *Feng Ch'eng* 豐 城 , and the various medical works. As all people have five senses[7] and four limbs, so all require gymnastics, pressure, and friction. Kung-fu divides itself into external actions and internal merit; everyone chooses their own kind. The ancients divided actions into twelve kinds and wrote the method to be followed in poetry, so that all might remember the rules laid down. All can do them, at all times, and everyone can understand them quick-ly and efficaciously.

There is no necessity here for claptrap and useless nonsense; the true and important object is to drive away or ward off disease and pro-cure long life. Belief in this plan will bring merit out of it. The doctrines of Lao Tzu, 老 子 , C-hih-sung Tzu 赤 松 子 ,[8] and Chung-li

---

[6][Ed. note: Moxibustion, the application of small burning cores of vege-table matter to the skin.]

[7]Eyes, ears, nose, mouth, and eyebrows; all the five senses must be in the head, the heavenly part of the human being, like high ministers close to the Emperor.

[8]The designation of a rain-priest in the time of Shen-nung.

Tzu, 鍾 離 子 [9] are not superior to the precepts of this book. If one can perform the exercises herein prescribed once or twice daily, the body will become strong and elastic, and no matter how many kinds of diseases one may have, all will vanish. Thus will the vital principle exist in adequate quantity, and life consequently prolonged. This is surely good, and on this account I have taken up my pen to write this preface.

[9]The first and greatest of the Eight Immortals in the time of the Chou dynasty (B.C. 1122–255), when he attained possession of the elixir of immortality.

DIAGRAM ILLUSTRATING THE
PHYSIOLOGY OF KUNG-FU

1. *T'ien-men* (heavenly door), the brow
2. *Ni-wan kung*, Ni-wan palace.
3. *Sui-hai-ku*, the occiput, marrow-sea, brain-sea.
4. *San chiao*, the three divisions or functional passages.
5. *Fei*, the lungs
6. *Hsin*, the heart.
7. *Hsin-pao-lo*, the pericardium.
8. *Kan*, the liver.
9. *Wei*, the stomach.
10. *P'i*, the spleen.
11. *Huang-t'ing tan-t'ien*, the inner *tan* of the yellow pavilion.
12. *Ta ch'ang*, the large intestines.
13. *Hsiao ch'ang*, the small intestines.
14. *Shen*, the kidneys.
15. *P'ang-kuang*, the bladder.
16. *Yü-ching shan* (pearly-elevated hill), 7th cervical vertebra.
17. *Chia-chi*, the dorsal vertebra.
18. *Wei-lü*, the os sacrum.
19. *Shang shui hsia huo wei chi chi chien yü lien lou chih hsia* (water above and fire below combine and are seen below the connecting "upper story"), *i.e.*, the *tan-t'ien* below the breast and epigastriam = the *lou* or upper story, according to the Taoists.
20. *Tan chung chen huo shang sheng* (the true fire in the *tan-t'ien* proceeds upwards).

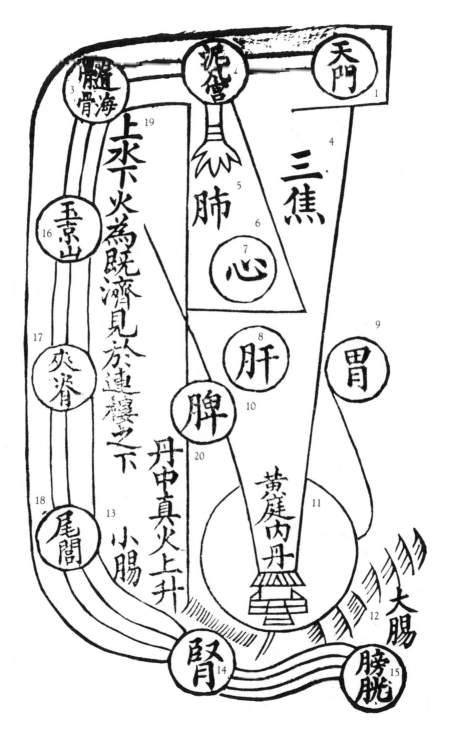

功夫 Old Works on Kung-Fu

The Taoist work *Tsun-sheng-pa-chien* 遵生八牋, in 20 books, was written by Kao-lien Shen-fu 高濂深甫 in 1591. The first and third prefaces are by the author, the second by Ch'ai Ying-nan 柴應楠. The work is divided into eight parts. Two books are occupied with the subject of Undivided Application; four with Seasonable Regimen, from which we have taken the Kung-fu for the Four Seasons; two with Rest and Pleasure; two with Prevention of Disease, from which we have taken the Eight Ornamental Sections; three with Eating, Drinking, and Clothing; three with Amusements in Retirement; two with Efficacious Medicines; and one with Examples of the Virtuous. The Contents form the twentieth volume. In the large list of drugs the poppy is mentioned only once, and among a list of prescriptions opium occurs only once, as an ingredient in a pill entitled The Great Golden Elixir.

This work is well-written; there is a sameness of language and illustration running through the works of this class. The more recent and cheaper books have been reproduced from the older works with minor changes and additions.

Another work, called *Hsing-ming-kuei-chih* 性命圭旨, is by an accomplished Taoist of the Sung dynasty named Yin Chen-jen 尹眞人; it is on the Government of the Inner Person. This is one of the most celebrated treatises on this art. It is in four volumes and treats at large of the principles and methods of practice; it is amply illustrated by plates. It was first printed in 1615, and another edition in a large and handsome style was issued about 1670. The first preface is by Li P'o 李樸, the second by Ch'ang Chi 常吉, the third by Tsou Yuan-piao 鄒元標, and the fourth by Yu T'ung 尤侗, all in the time of the K'anghsi emperor (1662–1723 A.D.).

The contents of this work are of the usual Taoist character: discourses on the Great Reason, Birth, Life, Death, the Elixir, the Absolute, Yin and Yang, Refining the Heart, etc. One chapter, entitled The Three Passes, Agreeing and Opposing, begins thus: "Reason (Tao) produced one; one produced two; two produced three and three produced the myriad things." Another chapter on the True and False, or the deflected and the perfect, begins with the great Tao producing heaven and earth.

This states that there are 3,600 Taoist methods, twenty-four sorts of the Great Elixir, and ninety-six sorts of outside doctrines.[1] There are numerous side sects but only one Golden Elixir Doctrine, which is the one and only perfect way. Outside this, there is no way of becoming Immortals and Buddhas. This is real; all else is empty and false. About sixty different sects who practice their doctrine are mentioned, hoping by these means to gain immortality. The list is said to be inexhaustible. Their methods are compared to looking through a tube at the panther (and seeing one spot only) or looking at heaven from the bottom of a well, the horizon in both cases being contracted and limited, for there is no panacea but the Golden Elixir, the Great Reason. The list, though intensely interesting and instructive, is too long to reproduce here.

Another work is called *Fu-shou-tan-shu* 福 壽 丹 書, or the Elixir of Happiness and Longevity, in six volumes, published in 1621. Hua-to's Five Animals are drawn from the first volume of this work, entitled *An-yang-p'ien* 安 養 篇, a Discourse on Peace and Nourishment. The second volume is termed *Yen-ling-p'ien* 延 齡 篇, a Treatise on Longevity; the Medicinal *Kung* are extracted from this volume. The remaining four volumes are entitled respectively *Fu-shih-p'ien* 服 食 篇, a collection of prescriptions on dress and food by Ying Yuan; *Ts'ai-pu-p'ien* 採 補 篇, by the same; *Hsaen-hsien-p'ien* 玄 脩 篇, ditto; and On Drugs, or *Ch'ing-yao-p'ien* 清 樂 篇 by Cheng Chih-ch'iao 鄭 之 僑.

Another work is termed *Tan-i-san-chüan* 丹 擬 三 卷, in six volumes, consisting of *T'ien-hsien-cheng-li* 天 仙 正 理 in two books by Pa-Tzu-yuan 巴 子 園, reprinted in the year 1801; one volume entitled *Fo-hsien-ho-tsung* 佛 仙 合 宗, a Harmony of Buddhism and Taoism, by Wu-Shen-yang in the reign of Wan-li (1572–1620 A.D.); and three volumes entitled *Wan-shou-hsien-shu* 萬 壽 仙 書, the same in import as the *Yen-ling-p'ien* or Treatise on Longevity. The first volume contains the Eight Ornamental Sections and the year's illustrations, in

---

[1][Ed. note: exoteric as opposed to esoteric teachings.]

every respect identical with those of the *Tsun-sheng-pa-chien*, except that the list of diseases which the exercise is designed to cure is very much briefer and more reasonable. We have followed the earlier work, from which this seems to have been copied. The miscellaneous illustrations in the second volume are identical with those in the *Yen-ling-p'ien* noticed above. The illustrations are inferior as works of art to the *Yen-ling-p'ien*, from which they have apparently been copied. My copy is, however, a cheap edition. The same volume also contains Hua-to's Five Animals and also Ch'en Hsi-i's Right and Left Sleeping Exercise, which occurs also in the volume on Prevention of Disease in the Future in the *Tsun-sheng-pa-chien*. The prefaces to most of these works are purely ornamental, conveying no exact truth or historical interest.

功夫 Kung-Fu for The Four Seasons

In the year's exercises, we must omit for lack of space all references to the time each day, which ranges from midnight to 7 A.M., when they are enjoined; also omitted are the numerous correlations with pulses, blood vessels, viscera, the Five Elements and their natures, the atmospheric influences—whether heavenly, earthly, or respiratory, the Eight Diagrams,[1] the Cyclical Signs,[2] the points of the compass, etc.

There are two exercises for each month, making twenty-four in all, arranged according to the twenty-four Solar Terms or periods of the year. These correspond to the days on which the sun enters the first and fifteenth degree of one of the zodiacal signs. An appropriate name is given to each of these, which we have retained, as they are in popular use. The exercises are arranged according to the four seasons, and each season is prefixed and suffixed with some animal representing the correlated viscera. These we have also retained for their excellency of design, and with the view of conveying an idea of the Chinese correspondencies. It will be observed that the Black Tiger and the Dragon occur very frequently in Taoist works. Charms also often accompany them; but, as this is a wide subject and has a special form of treatment, it is omitted here.

In the medicinal exercises which follow, I have given the prescriptions attached to them, as they throw some light upon the Chinese materia medica and mode of preparing drugs, the nature of their recipes, etc. Included in the chapters on *Seasonable Regimen*, referred to further

[1][Ed. note: The eight trigrams of the *I Ching*.]
[2][Ed. note: The Twelve Earthly Branches and Ten Celestial Stems, which are combined to form a cycle of sixty used in designating successive days or years.]

on, are found prescriptions ascribed to Huang-ti for the cure or prevention of diseases of the viscera, which are omitted. The spring governs birth; summer, growth; autumn, harvesting; and winter, storage. For each period and for each viscus, the various things that regulate and assist are given, what is indicated and what contra-indicated, with all matters that ought to be attended to.

The liver is the viscus which stands at the head of the three months of spring. It is represented as a dragon. [See illustration below.] The name of its spirit is "Dragon Smoke;" its appellation is "Containing Brightness." The form of the liver is that of a dragon; it stores up the soul; it

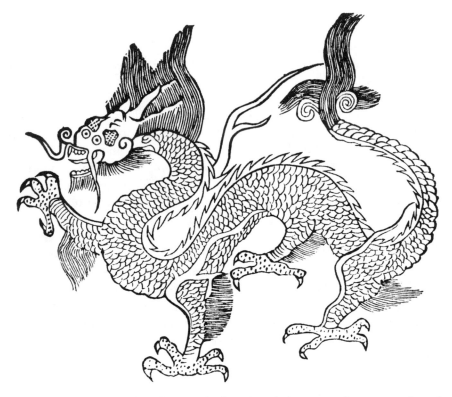

resembles a hanging bottle-gourd of a whitish brown colour; it is placed below the heart, a little nearer the back. The right has four lobes, the left three lobes; its pulse emerges from the end of the thumb. The liver is the mother of the heart and the son of the kidneys.

To repair and nourish it, during the first half of the three months one must sit facing the east, knock the teeth 3 times, shut the breath and inspire 9 times; breathe the south air, take in 9 mouthfuls and swallow 9 times. [Certain medicines are also ordered.]

The *kung* to direct the liver for the spring three months is to press the two hands on the shoulders equally; slowly press the body right and left each three times. It can also be done by clasping or interlocking the two hands, turning the palms and dorsa alternately to the chest 3 x 5 (15) times. This will cure obstruction of the liver from vicious wind and poisonous air and prevent disease from developing.

These exercises must be incessantly attended to morning and evening in the spring, without missing even one day; with the heart set upon it, the cure is complete. After one has driven out the corrupt air and the eyes are fixed and closed, open them only a little, and then puff out the air slowly and by little; the cure of a flushed face and flow of tears will be effected.

1. For the Solar Term of the First Month, or "Beginning of Spring"

Hands folded, press the thigh; turn the body; twist the neck towards the right and left alternately 3 x 5 (15) times; knock the teeth, respire, gargle [as it were the air in the mouth], and swallow 3 times. For the cure of rheumatism and obstructions; pain in the neck, shoulders, ear, back, elbow, and arm.

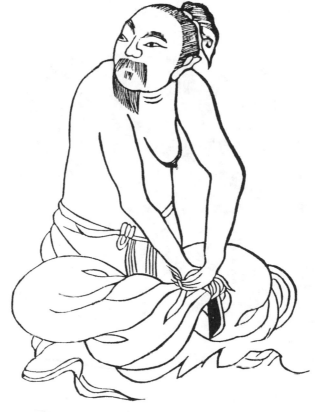

2. For the Middle of the First Month, or "Rain Water"

Hands folded, press the thigh; turn the neck 3 x 5 (15) times, etc., as in the first exercise. For the cure of obstruction and storing up of vicious poison in the Three Divisions; difficult deglutition, deafness, and pain of the eyes.

3. For the Solar Term of the Second Month, or "Waking of Insects"[3]

Close the fists tightly; turn the neck; move the elbows like the wings (of a bird) 5 x 6 (30) times; draw them backwards and forwards; tap the

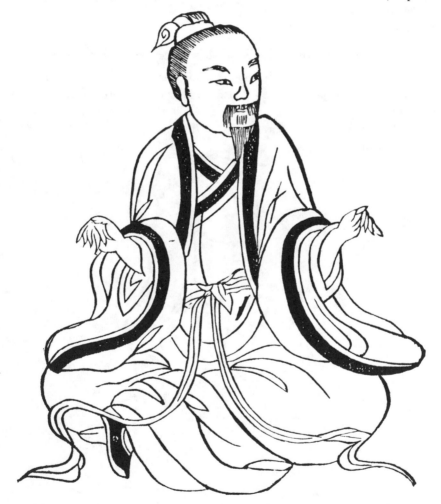

[3]Animals that have secreted themselves all winter are supposed to come out on this day.

teeth 6 x 6 (36) times; inspire and swallow 3 x 3 (9) times. To cure obstructions of the loins [lumbago], back, lungs, and stomach; dryness of the mouth, yellowness of the eyes; rheumatism of the head; toothache, darkness of vision, intolerance of light, loss of smell, and boils all over the body.

4. For the Middle of the Second Month, or "Spring Equinox"

Extend the hands; turn the head to the right and left 6 x 7 (42) times; knock the teeth 6 x 6 (36); inspire and swallow 3 x 3 (9). To cure weakness and the vicious poison of the chest [consumption], shoulders, back, and small blood vessels; toothache, feverishness, deafness or earache; pain of the shoulders, elbow, upper arm, and back.

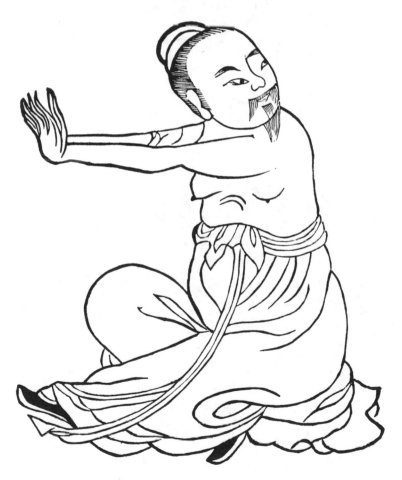

5. For the Solar Term of the Third Month, or "Pure Brightness"

Change hands, right and left, as if drawing a bow, each 7 x 8 (56) times; knock the teeth; respire—taking in the outside pure air to displace the foul air from within—and swallow the saliva, each 3 times. To cure the weakness and vicious air of the loins, kidneys, intestines, and stomach; painful deglutition; deaf and painful ears; pain of the neck and inability to turn it; pain in the shoulder; painful arm; and weakness of the loins.

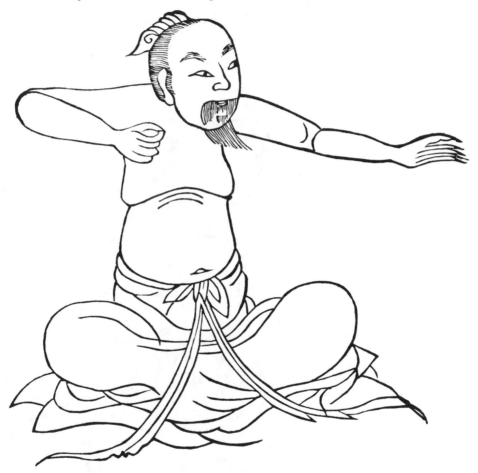

6. For the Middle of the Third Month, or "Corn Rain"

Sitting evenly, alternately raise the right and left hand as if supporting something; and alternately with the right and left [hand] cover the breasts, each 5 x 7 (35) times, etc. To cure blood obstruction in the spleen and stomach; yellowness of the eyes; bleeding of the nose; cheeks, neck and arm.

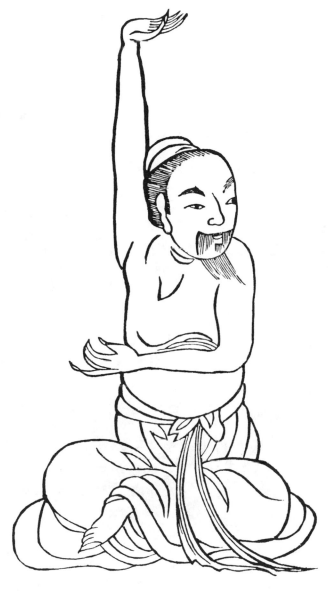

Each exercise concludes invariably with the phrase *t'u na yen yeh* 吐 納 嚥 液, which we have translated *respire and swallow the saliva* so many times. The word *t'u* refers to the air coming out of the mouth softly and slowly (expiration); *na* refers to its entering by the nose (inspiration) also slowly and continuously. The expression is equivalent to breathing out the foul and sniffing in the pure air. The repetition of the phrase is omitted.

The air of expiration moves the Heavenly Stems and the air of inspiration the Earthly Branches.

The name of the spirit of the gall bladder is "Glorious Dragon," and its appellation "Majestic Brightness." Its form is that of a tortoise coiled round by a serpent; its resemblance is to a suspended gourd; its colour is a green-purple; it is placed in the middle of the liver.

Its *kung* is to sit upright; place the two soles of the feet together; raise the head; take hold of the ankles with the hands and move the feet 3 x 5 (15) times. Or with the two hands press the ground; straighten the body; and add force to the loins and back 3 x 5 (15) times. In this way, the vicious air and poisonous wind can be driven out.

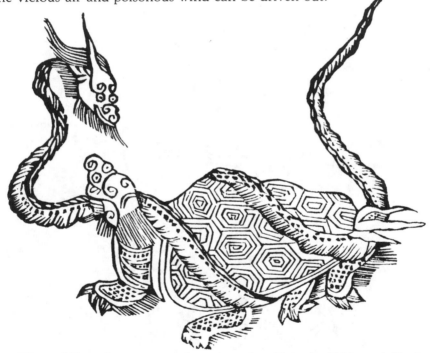

Then follow the summer three months—Fourth, Fifth and Sixth. The period starts with a picture of the heart. The name of its spirit is "Great Red;" its designation is "Guarding the Soul;" its form is like "the Scarlet Bird" (the fancy name of a position in geomancy); as the Red Ruler, it stores up the spirit. It resembles the lotus turned upside down; in colour, it is like white reflected on brown; it is placed in the middle of the lungs above the liver, one inch below the apex of the ensiform cartilage (in Chinese the aperture called the "dove's tail"). The pulse of the heart issues from the end of the left middle finger, at the aperture termed "the communicating centre."

In order to direct the heart into a right course, sit straight, with both hands clenched, and with strength ram down alternately the right and left hand each 5 x 6 (30) times. Also, raise one hand aloft in space as if supporting a picul of rice, right and left alternately. Also, clasp both hands and place the foot within the clasped hands, each 5 x 6 (30) times, during which period let the breath be held, to drive out all diseases caused by vicious wind in the heart and thorax. This exercise is to be performed for a long time, with the eyes shut, the saliva swallowed 3 times, and the teeth knocked 3 times. Afterwards *hem* slowly. Whatever grief may be in the heart or ulcers in the mouth will be cured. Or, sitting upright, throw both fists forward (as if fighting) and bring them back 6 times.

Two additional exercises for directing the heart are given as follows: *First*, sitting upright, body inclined, use strength in this position like a hill supporting a hill. In this way, sit, using force to drive out the vicious wind of the loins and spine, to make pervious the five viscera and six *fu*,

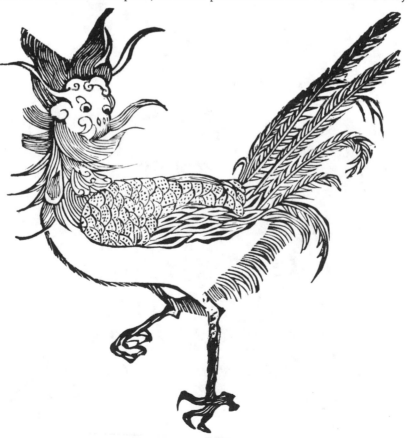

to disperse foot vapours (gout), to tone the heart, and to strengthen the system; do it the same on the right and left sides.

The *second* method is to press the stomach with one hand, and the raise the other hand upwards, using all your strength as if supporting a stone, and retain the breath; do the same on both sides, to dispel the poisonous wind of the ribs, to cure the heart, and cause the blood and pulses to circulate and harmonize.

When the seven apertures of the heart are all open, the Chinese assert attainment of the highest intelligence. With a moderate amount of wisdom, only five openings are pervious; in the case of the intensely stupid, all the openings are blocked up, and no air passes through. The heart is the son of the liver and mother of the spleen.

In the beginning of the Fourth and Fifth months, early in the morning, face the south and sit straight; bump the teeth 9 times; gargle the saliva in the mouth 3 times; think silently; draw the south air into the mouth and swallow 3 times, hold the breath, and take 30 inspirations after each such holding, and so fill up and replace the vicious air.

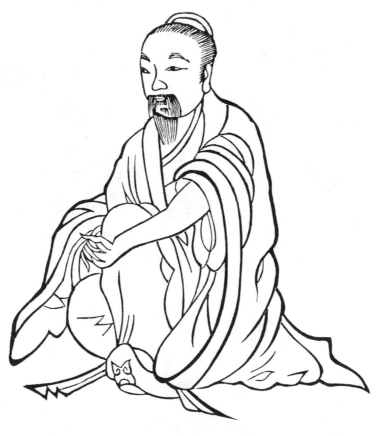

7. For the Solar Term of the Fourth Month, or "Beginning of Summer"

Breath closed and eyes shut, turn and change the hands, and press them on the knees each 5 x 7 (35) times, etc. To cure wind and dampness collected in the *ching-lo* or network of small blood vessels, swollen and painful arms and axillae, hot palms of the hands.

8. For the Middle of the Fourth Month, or "Small Full"

One hand is raised as if holding something up, one hand pressed down, right and left each 3 x 5 (15) times, etc. To cure obstructions in the liver and lungs of the usual characters [*i.e.*, the vitiated air and poison which

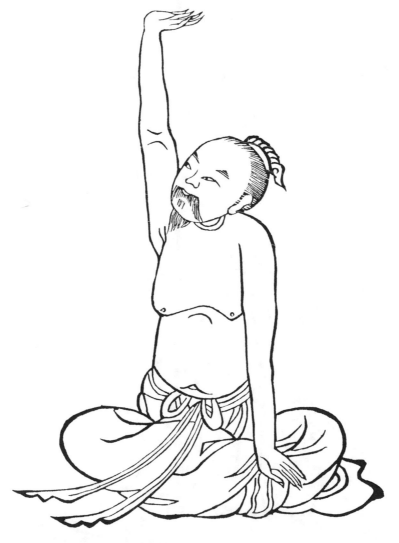

has become stagnant and refuses to disperse], fullness of the thorax and ribs, pain and palpitation of the heart, flushing of the face, yellow eyes, sad heart, pain and fear, hot palms of the hands.

9. For the Solar Term of the Fifth Month, or "Sprouting Seeds"

(Although the figure is standing, the instruction is sitting. The character for sitting (*tso*) seems, however, to indicate the passing of a season in

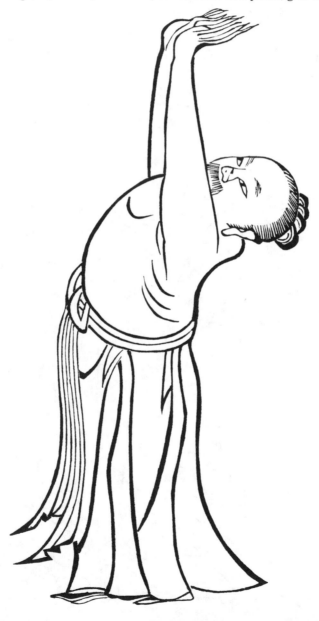

such exercises, just as *hsing-kung* 行 功 refers to the carrying out of the same; the latter expression occurs almost invariably in the body of the instructions, while the other 坐 forms the title or introduction.) The body is thrown back, both hands raised aloft as if supporting something, and great force is used with both right and left in raising up [the supposed weight] 5 x 7 (35) times. Fix the breath and perform the remainder as usual. To cure weakness of the loins and kidneys, dryness in swallowing, painful heart and ribs, yellow eyes, thirst, hot body and painful thighs, painful head and neck, red face, cough and expectoration upwards, leakage downwards (diarrhea), passage of wind, emission of semen.

10. For the Middle of the Fifth Month, or "Summer Solstice"

Kneel; stretch the hands; interlock the fingers and bend them over the foot; change the feet right and left each 5 x 7 (35) times, etc. To cure obstructed wind and undispersed damp [rheumatism]; painful knees, ankles, arms, kidneys, loins, and spine; and heaviness of the body.

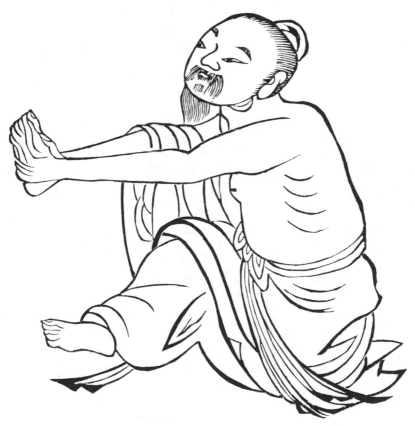

11. For the Solar Term of the Sixth Month, or "Slight Heat"

Press the two hands to the ground; bend one foot under the body; stretch out the other with force 3 x 5 (15) times, etc. To cure rheumatism of the legs, knees, thighs, and loins; fullness of the lungs with excessive flow of phlegm; asthma, cough, pain in the middle of the sternum, violent sneezing, abdominal distension and pain to the right of the navel; contracted hands [arthritis], heavy body, loss of memory, whooping cough, prolapsus ani, weakness of the wrist, inconstant joy and anger.

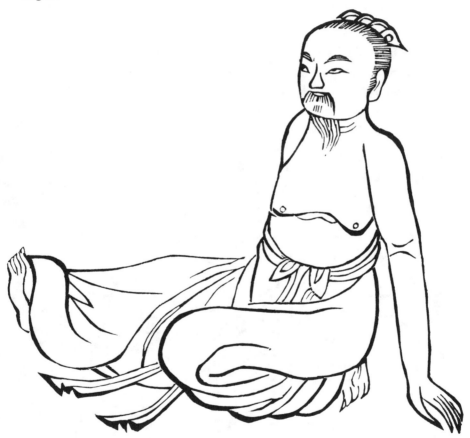

12. For the Middle of the Sixth Month, or "Great Heat"

Sit all in a heap on the ground; twist the head toward the shoulders, and look like a tiger to the right and left each 3 x 5 (15) times, etc. To cure rheumatism of the head, neck, chest, and back; cough and asthma;

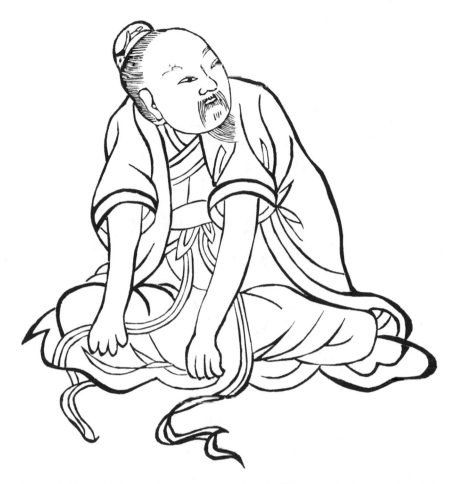

thirst dullness [taking pleasure in nothing]; fullness of chest; pain of the arm, hot palms of the hands, pain above the navel or in the shoulder and back, cold and hot perspiration, inclination to grief and crying.

For the last half of the Sixth Month, the *kung-fu* is to sit quite straight; extend the fingers upwards, then bend them backwards; perform this 3 times, then bend them to the front in the same way, in front and behind alike. To cure the loins, spine, and feet, and to disperse the vicious air of the bladder.

The spleen is called "Constantly Present;" designation, the "Soul's Residence;" in form, phoenix-like. It secretes the soul, resembles an upturned basin; its colour is like white reflected on yellow; it covers the centre above the navel, in front covers the stomach horizontally; its pulse issues from the side of the end of the left foot's big toe just at the corner of the nail.

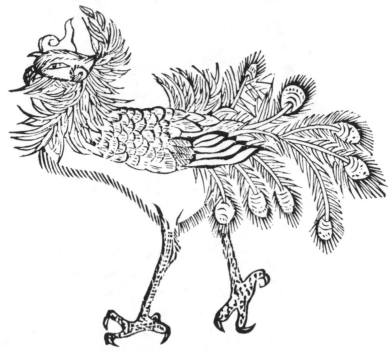

During the Sixth Month, the following exercise is given as "directing into the right courses." Extend one foot; bring both hands to the front, and let them draw the feet 3 x 5 (15) times. Also, kneel, both hands grasping the earth; turn the head, using force look like a tiger 3 x 5 (15) times. This exercise can drive away the rheumatism which obstructs the spleen and promotes digestion.

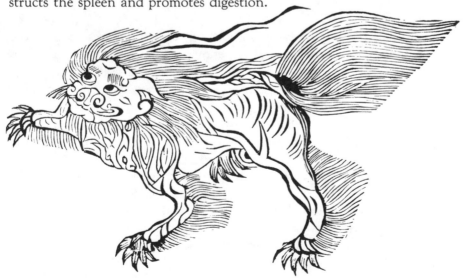

The tiger appears as the illustration of the lungs in the *kung* beginning the Autumnal Three Months. Its spirit's name is "Truly Beautiful," and its designation "Empty Completeness." It is like a tiger and secretes the soul. It resembles the suspended bell (*ching*) of the Buddhists; its colour is like white reflected on red; it is placed above the heart, opposite the chest, and is of six lobes. Its pulse issues from the inside of the end of the left thumb.

The *kung* for the Seventh, Eighth, and Ninth Months is: with both hands grasp the ground; contract the body; bend the spine; and raise the body 3 times, to disperse the vicious wind of the lungs and the old injuries that are collected there. Also turn the fist and beat the back with the left and right hands, each 3 times, to drive out the enclosed poisonous air in the thorax; and, after having done this for a long time, shut the eyes, knock the teeth, and rise.

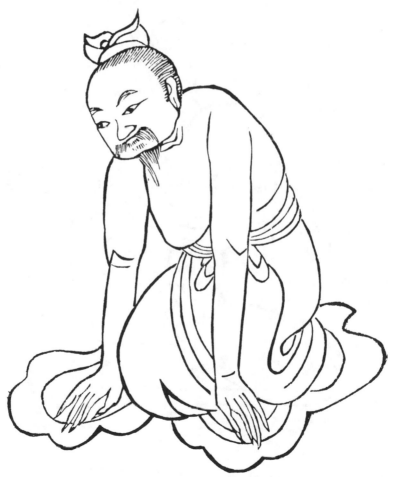

13. For the Solar Term of the Seventh Month, or "Beginning of Autumn"

Both hands to the ground, contract the body; close the breath; raise up the body in a jerking manner 7 x 8 (56) times, etc. To fill up the empty (weak) and injured parts; to dispel the air of the loins and kidneys collected there, for painful heart and ribs and inability to turn the body; hot outside of the foot; headache, painful jaws, protruding eyes, swollen and painful sternum and armpits, cold perspiration.

14. For the Middle of the Seventh Month, or "Stopping of Heat"

Turn the head to the right and left; raise the head; turn the two hands and beat the back each 5 x 7 (35) times, etc. To cure rheumatism; pain

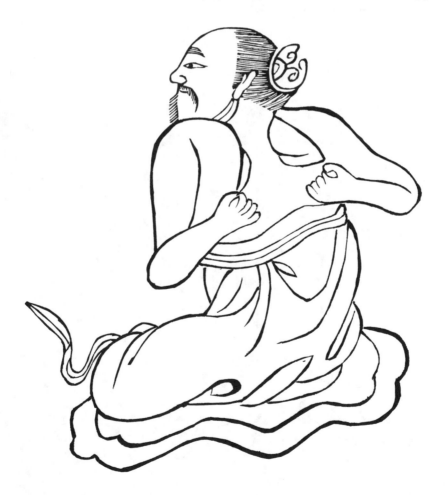

of the shoulder, back, chest, ribs, thighs, knees, small blood vessels, outside of the leg and ankle; pain of the various joints; cough, asthma, shortness of breath, thirst.

15. For the Solar Term of the Eighth Month, or "White Dew"

Seated upright, press the two hands on the knees; turn the head, pushing and stretching it each 3 x 5 (15) times, etc. To cure rheumatism of the loins and back, lips deepened in colour, swollen neck, retching, insanity, flushed face.

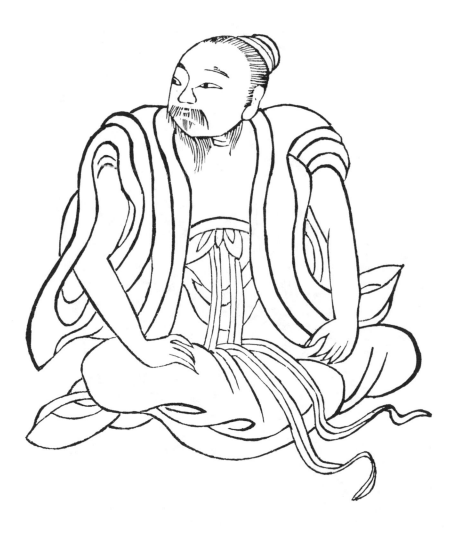

16. For the Middle of the Eighth Month, or "Autumnal Equinox"

Sitting cross-legged, both hands covering the ears, turn sideways to the right and left 3 x 5 (15) times, etc. To cure rheumatism of the ribs, loins, thighs, knees, and ankles; distension of the abdomen with rumbling of air; a feeling as if air were colliding with the breasts; painful thighs, legs and ankles; incontinence of urine, inability to turn the thighs, very rapid digestion; cold stomach, great thirst.

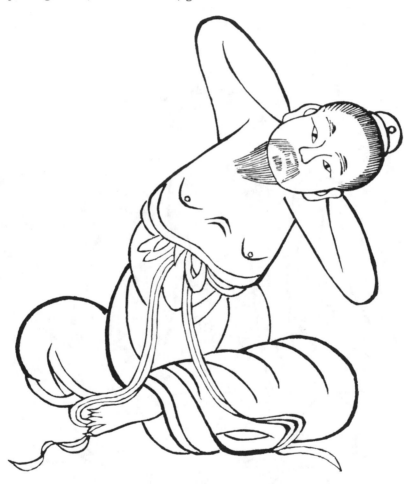

17. For the Solar Term of the Ninth Month, or "Cold Dew"

Sitting upright, raise both arms; jerk up the body as if supporting something, right and left 5 x 7 (35) times, etc. To cure all sorts of vicious wind, cold, and damp; pain of the ribs, neck, loins, and spine; headache, hemorrhoids, insanity, yellowness of eyes.

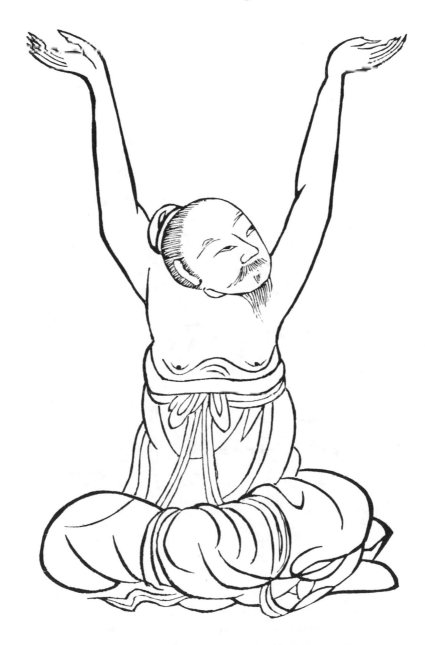

18. For the Middle of the Ninth Month, or "Frost's Descent"

Seated even, extend both hands and seize the feet; accompanying this exercise, use strength in the middle of the feet, then relax and withdraw the hands 5 x 7 (35) times, etc. To cure wind and damp that has entered the loins; inability to extend and flex the feet and thighs; painful joints; painful lower part of the leg, back, loins, pelvis, thighs, and knees; muscular paralysis, the small abdomen distended and painful, cold tendons, gout, hemorrhoids, prolapsus ani.

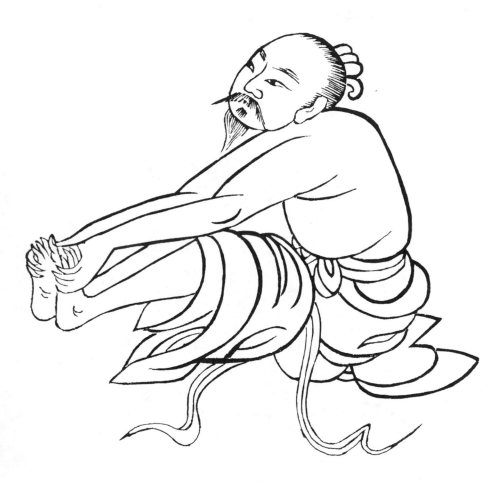

The kidneys form the illustration at the beginning of the last three months of the year, which is as follows: The name of its spirit is "The Water Spirit," and its designation "Nourishing Infants." Its form is that of a yellow deer with two heads. It stores up the will. It resembles a round stone, is of two colours like white silk reflected on purple. It is placed opposite the navel, and lies in close contact with the lumbar spine. The left kidney is the real one, and mates with the five viscera. The right kidney is called the *Ming-men* 命 門 or "Gate of Life," and in the male secretes the semen, In the female the fetal membrane. The pulse of the kidney issues from the middle of the soles of the feet.

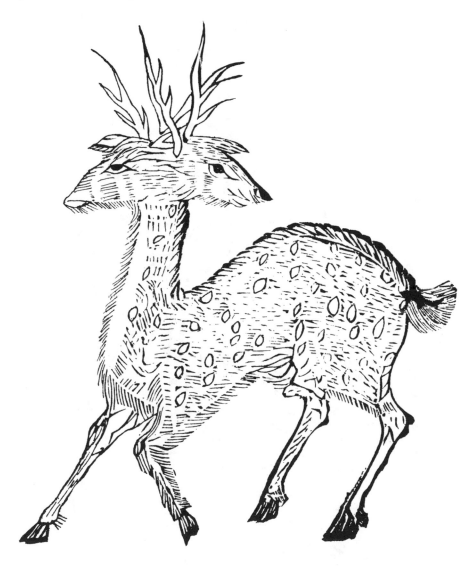

19. For the Solar Term of the Tenth Month, or "Beginning of Winter"

Seated upright, one hand on the knee, one hand grasping the elbow, change right and left and support the right and left 3 x 5 (15) times, etc. To cure a deficiency of saliva; nausea and hiccough; indigested fecal motions; headache, deafness, swollen jaws; red, swollen and painful eyes; sense of fullness and depression in abdomen and ribs and the four extremities; vertigo, painful pupils.

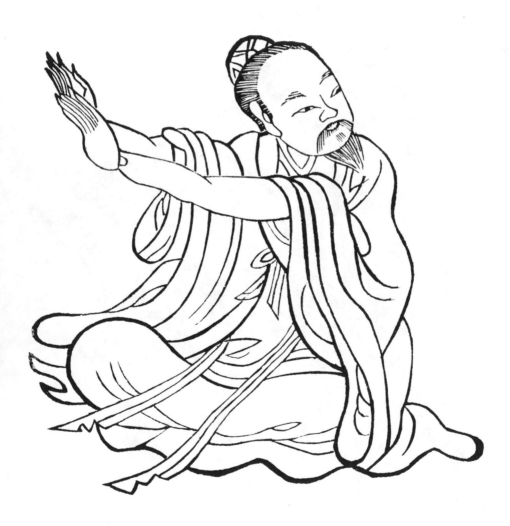

20. For the Middle of the Tenth Month, or "Slight Snow"

Place one hand on the knee, the other grasping the elbow, right and left using force 3 x 5 (15) times, etc. To cure a wife's enlargement of the small abdomen and a husband's hernia; incontinence of urine, swelling of the joints, contraction of the tendons, small *membrum virile*; five sorts of gonorrhea [wind, fire, cold, poison, damp]; diarrhea, fear, fullness of the chest, asthma of the lower ribs.

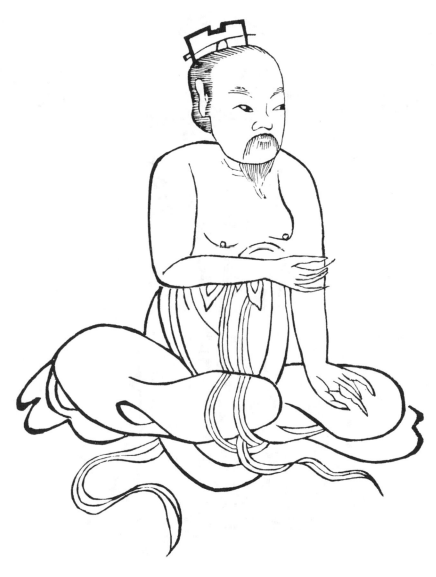

21. For the Solar Term of the Eleventh Month, or "Great Snow"

Stand straight, the knees extended, both hands to the right and left as if supporting the two feet; stamp right and left, each 5 x 7 (35) times, etc. To cure wind and dampness of the feet and knees; heat of the mouth, dryness of the tongue, swelling of the throat; jaundice, hunger with inability to eat; cough, asthma, fear.

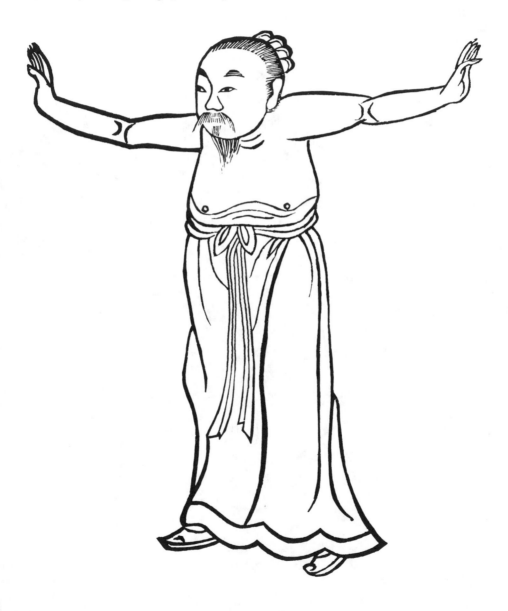

22. For the Middle of the Eleventh Month, or "Winter Solstice"

Sitting evenly, extend both feet; clench the two hands, and press both knees; with extreme force perform this with the right and left 3 x 5 (15) times, etc. To cure cold and damp of the hands, feet, spine, and thighs; pain of the lower ribs between the shoulders and the middle of the thighs; fullness of the thorax; distension of the abdomen; cough; loins that are cold like water and swollen; air below the navel that is not harmonious; little belly [below the navel] that is very painful; diarrhea, swollen feet, dysentery.

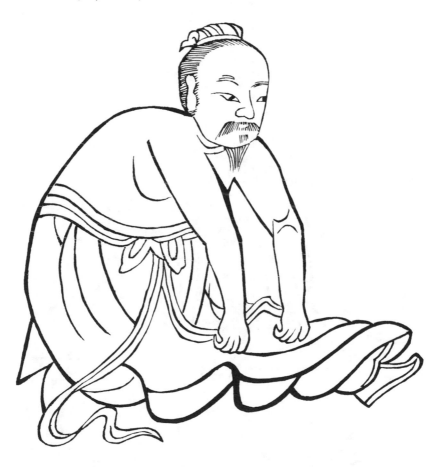

23. For the Solar Term of the Twelvth Month, or "Slight Cold"

Sitting upright, one hand pressing the foot, the other raised aloft as if supporting something, turn the head and change [the hands] alternately; use great force 3 x 5 (15) times, etc. To cure the air stored up in the arteries and veins; retching and vomiting, painful stomach, distended abdomen; fullness of thorax, failing appetite, sighing, great heaviness of body, grief, diarrhea, suppression of urine, jaundice; the five diarrheas of five colours, dry mouth, indolence, desire to lie down, lack of appetite.

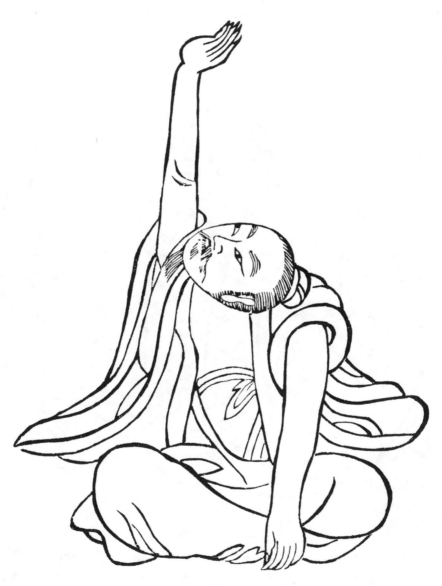

24. For the Middle of the Twelvth Month, or "Great Cold"

Both hands thrown behind, kneeling with one foot extended straight out; with one foot use force right and left alternately each 3 x 5 (15) times, etc. To cure the storage of all sorts of influences in the small network of blood vessels; a root of the tongue that is hard, painful, and unable to move; inability to move the body or to lie down; inability to stand great expenditure of strength; swollen thighs; painful pelvis, thighs, legs, feet, and back; distension of the abdomen, rumbling in the intestines, indigested food causing diarrhea; feet unable to be pulled together in order to walk; the nine openings that are impervious.

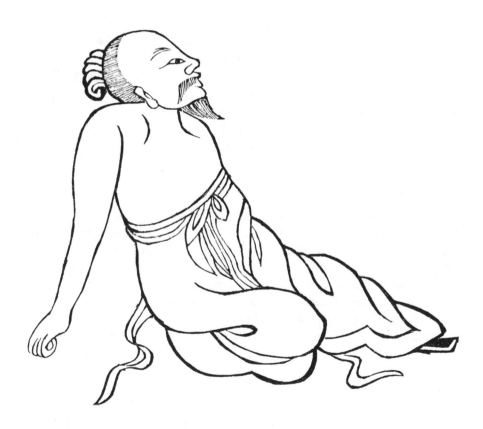

功夫 The Eight Ornamental Sections

This name has been handed down by the sages of antiquity, and hence the eight illustrations. The object aimed at is to prevent the entrance of bad air, to obtain clearness in dreams and sleep, to shut out cold and heat from the body, and to prevent disease from gaining a lodgment. The time when the exercises are enjoined to be carried out is after the third watch [11 P.M. to 1 A.M.] and before noon, as this period agrees with the creation of heaven and earth, and also with their fixed series of diurnal revolutions;[1] the blood and air cannot stop, but must proceed also in their revolutions, and this is in accordance with the principles of the Eight Diagrams, which has excellent reason on its side.

The idea in the expression "to close the fist tightly" has not been deeply investigated. Not only must the eyes be closed and see one's own eyes, and thus the heart shut to the external world, but when one is sitting cross-legged, the left heel must be so flexed as to buttress the movable place [perineum] below the root of the *membrum virile* of the kidney, so as to prevent the leakage of semen.

In performing this *kung*, it is not absolutely necessary to do it at the periods specified. Any time of the day when the body is at leisure and the heart unoccupied will do equally well. To use the exercise much or little must be left to each person's discretion. If, however, persons will abide by the after midnight and before noon arrangements, and if at these periods they should have no leisure, what then? Those who wish to learn *Tao* cannot but understand this. [Such is the native introduction to these sections. It will be observed that they are prophylactic.]

[1][Ed. note: The history of the universe (macrocosm) is mirrored in the progression of each day (microcosm), so that each watch corresponds to a particular part of the universal cycle.]

1. Knocking the Teeth and Collecting the Spirits

Bump the teeth and assemble the spirits 36 times. Let the two hands embrace the *K'un-lun*[2] [the head] and beat the "Heavenly Drum" [the occiput] 24 times.

Note: The eyes must first be shut and the heart dark [*i.e.*, in Taoist phraseology, sit cross-legged], the fists must be tightly closed and the heart at rest, and both hands placed behind the vertex [of the head];

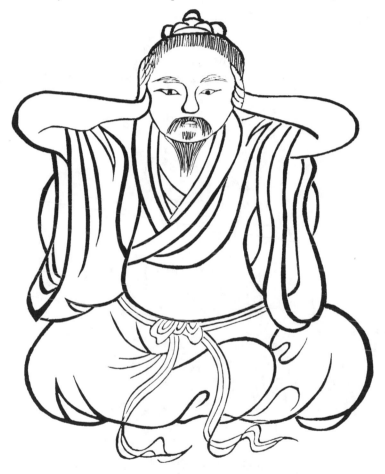

[2]A mountain in Central Asia, widely celebrated in Chinese legends, especially in ancient fable and Taoist mythology. The cosmogonists and mystics elevated it to the position of the central mountain of the earth, or as we say now "the roof of heaven," and the source of the "four great rivers," also the residence of the Queen of the Immortals. Innumerable marvels are related of this mountain, with its trees of pearls, jade-stone, and immortality. The appropriation of the name of this mountain to the head is, therefore, not out of place.

then [perform] 9 respirations such that the ears will not hear, and after-wards respire, still inaudible to the ears; then sound the "Heavenly Drum" 24 times; afterwards knock the teeth and assemble the spirits; then both hands with their palms must cover the ears, and the forefinger is to press upon the middle finger; the back of the brain is to be tapped right and left each 24 times. [The occiput is also sometimes termed the "Jade Pillow."]

2. Shaking the "Heavenly Pillar"

The right and left hand shake the "heavenly pillar" 24 times each.

Note: First close the fists tightly, then move the head once right and left; look at the shoulder and upper arm while following the movement 24 times.

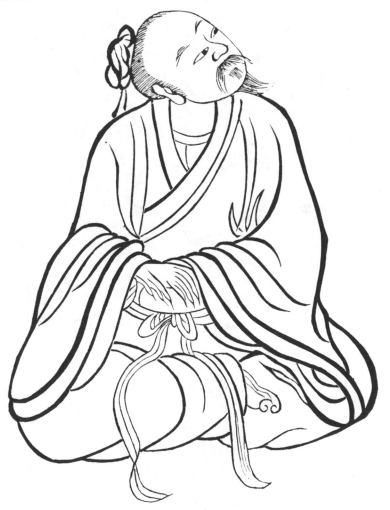

3. The Tongue Exciting, Gargling and Swallowing the Saliva

Let the tongue stir up the palate right and left 36 times, gargle 36 times, divide [the saliva thus produced] into 3 mouthfuls, and swallow [the saliva] as if it were a hard thing; afterwards the "fire" (inflammation) will go.

Note: Let the tongue excite the mouth, teeth, right and left cheeks; when the saliva has been thus produced, gargle; when the mouth is full, swallow it. The tongue is the "red dragon," the saliva is the "divine water," and the swallowing of the three mouthfuls must imitate the sound *ku-ku* 汩 汩 [the sound of gurgling water].

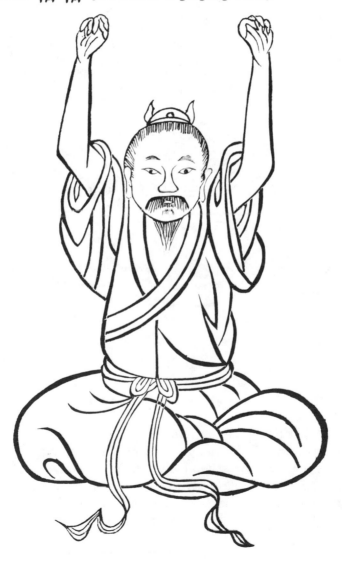

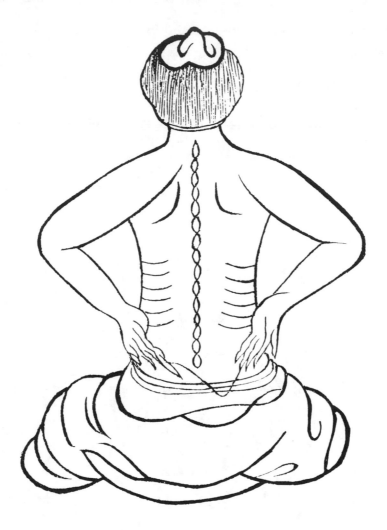

4. Rubbing the Kidneys

With both hands rub the court or hall of the kidneys [the loins] 36 times, the more the better. [*T'ang* 堂 , *chia* 家 , and *fu* 府 are indifferently used, and, when applied to the viscera, denote their residence].

Note: Close the respiration, rub the hands until warm, then rub the kidneys according to the number of times already mentioned; afterwards draw back the hands and close the fists tightly. Again shut the breath, reflect, use the fire of the heart and burn [heat] the *tan-tien* [navel]; when you feel that it has become very hot, then use the subsequent method. In the expression "the dragon going and the tiger fleeing," the saliva represents the dragon, and the air [of respiration] the tiger. In closing the breath and rubbing the hands warm, the nose first inspires the pure air, and then the respiration is closed; after a little, the hands are rubbed quickly until they become quite hot, then slowly let the nose give exit to the air. To rub the back *ching men* 精 門 [*i.e.*, semen door] means the external kidney behind the loins [as explained by the Chinese]. When the joining of the hands in rubbing is finished, withdraw the hands and grasp the fists firmly [as before]. Again shutting off the air, think of the fire as burning the "wheel of the navel." This refers to the *tan-tien*, and using the "heart fire" to think it down to the heating of the *tan-tien*.

5. Winding the Single Pulley

With the right and left [hands], turn the single pulley 36 times.

Note: First bend the head and move the left shoulder 36 times, then the right also 36 times.

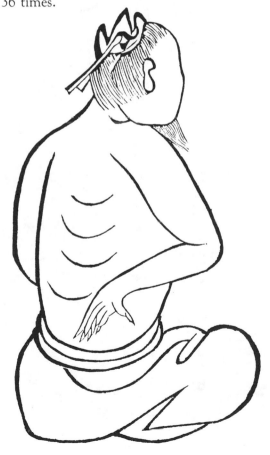

6. Winding the Double Pulley

Thirty-six times.

Note: Move the two shoulders like a pendulum 36 times. Bend the head, move the shoulders, think the fire from the *tan-tien* upwards by the "double pass" [one of the acupuncture apertures in the back] to the brain, the nose introducing the pure air; then close for a brief period, and extend the feet.

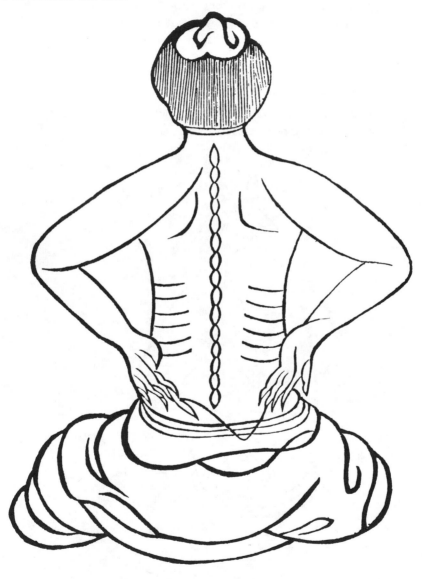

7. Pressing the Vertex

Rub the two hands together, and after five *hems* [voluntary half-coughs; in Chinese, *k'o* 呵], interlace the hands and support Heaven, and then press the vertex each 9 times.

    Note: Interlock the hands and raise them aloft to support the Void 3 or 9 times.

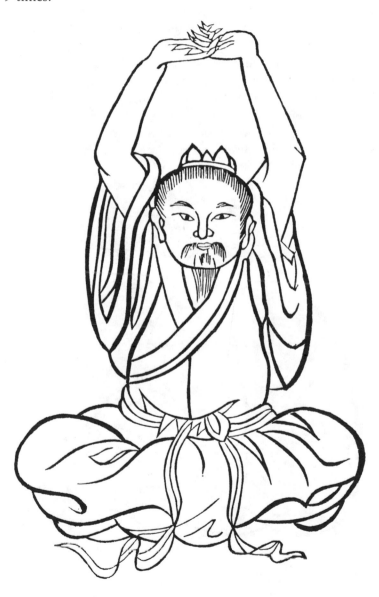

8. Grasping the Hook

Let the two hands take the form of a hook; advance them to the front; grasp the soles of the feet 12 times; again withdraw the feet and sit upright.

Note: Bring both hands to the front; clasp the soles of the feet 12 times; re-collect the feet and sit upright. Wait until the saliva in the mouth is produced, then gargle and swallow according to the number of times already indicated; move the shoulders and body 24 times, and also [perform] the pulley exercise [termed the "river cart"] 24 times; think the fire of the *tan-tien* from below upwards, and burn [heat] the body. At the time of thinking, the mouth and nose must be closed for a very little. Wait until the saliva is produced in the mouth; if it fails, then re-excite it, gargle and swallow according to the former method. When the "divine water" is swallowed 9 times, and the gurgling sound produced, the pulses become harmonized and regulated.

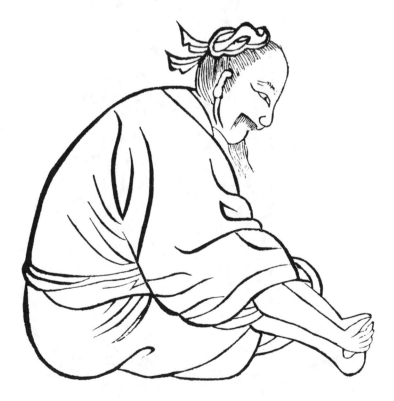

The Five Animals

These figures for the cure of disease by perspiration were designed by the celebrated surgeon Hua-to of the Han dynasty (2nd century A.D.), who was well-versed in the secrets of Taoism. He was wondrously skilled in acupuncture, and some of his surgical operations are of a very marvellous description. He was the first to use anaesthetics in scraping the poison from the arm of Kuan-ti, the god of war and patron of the Ch'ing dynasty. If one's body is not in health and peace, the performance of these five figures will produce perspiration and cure the disease and discomfort.

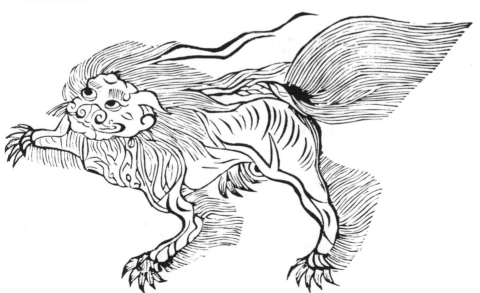

1. The Tiger

Close the breath, bend the head, close the fists tightly, and assume the severe form of a tiger. The two hands are slowly to lift a supposed weight of 1000 catties; the breath is to be retained until the body is upright, then swallowed and carried down into the abdomen. This is to cause the "divine air" [animal spirits, energy] to proceed from above downwards and produce in the abdomen a sound like thunder. To be done some 7 times. By this sort of movement, the air and pulses of the body will be harmonized and the hundred [all] diseases prevented from being produced.

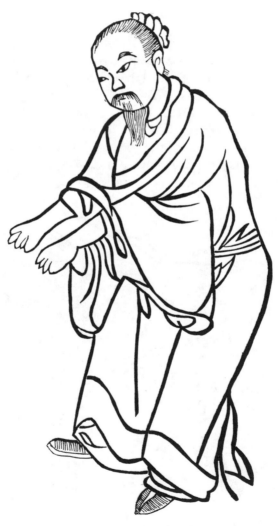

2. The Bear

Assume the form of a bear, incline the body slightly to the side, swing it to the right and left, place one foot in front and one behind, and stand fast. Use the air until the ribs on the two sides and the joints all resound. Also, move the strength of the loins to remove the swelling [?] some 3 to 5 times. This will relax and tranquillize the tendons and bones. This is also the method for nourishing the blood.

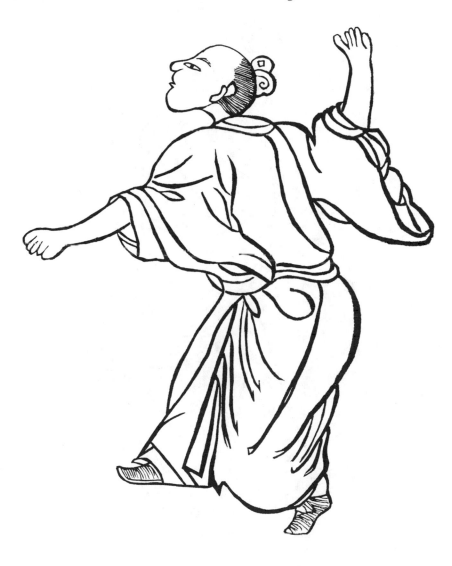

3. The Deer

Shut the breath, bend the head, close the fists tightly, turn the head like a deer viewing its tail; the body even, contract the shoulders, stand on tip-toe, stamp on the heel, and including the "heavenly pillar" [the neck] the entire body will move. Do it some 3 times, or once each day will also do. To do it once, on getting out of bed in the morning is the best [time] of all.

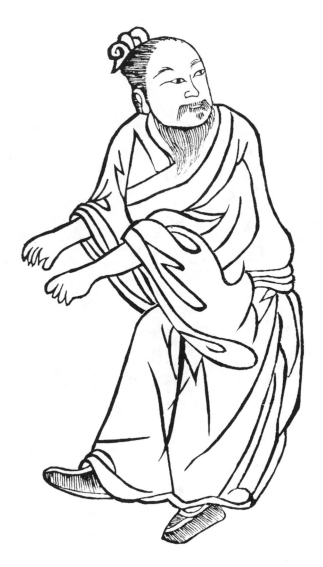

4. The Monkey

Stop the breath; assume the form of a monkey climbing a tree, one hand as it were holding some fruit, one foot raised; turn the body on the heel of one foot and cause the "divine air" to revolve,[1] carrying it into the abdomen until you feel perspiration is exuding, and then it is finished.

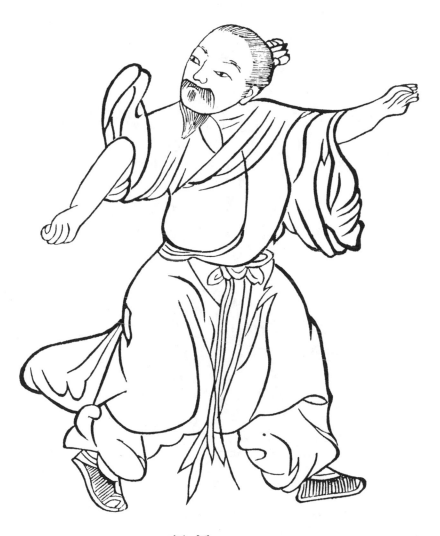

[1]The expression *yun-ch'i* 運 氣 occurs in almost every exercise. In fact, without this there is, properly speaking, no *kung*. It is the very essence of the art, and the greatest stress is laid upon it. The human is considered a "little heaven." The pure air is inspired, and, by one's swallowing with effort, it is carried down to the navel or *tan-tien*—an imaginary spot one inch below the

5. The Bird

Close the breath, assume the form of a bird flying, raise the head, inspire the air of the coccyx, and cause it to ascend to the hollow of the vertex [head]; let the two hands assume in front [the attitude of] reverence (or worship), raise the head [so as to have the face upwards], and go out to meet the spirit and break the vertex [*i.e.*, open the brain, as it were, to receive it].

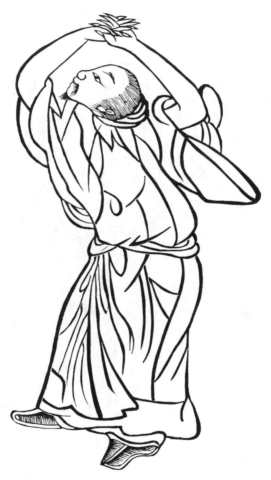

navel—and thence to the coccyx, where there is an aperture which in young persons is pervious but in old persons is filled up with fat; thence up the back, past the "double barrier" to the occiput; then over the vertex to the "heavenly door" (the brow); and finally it finds egress by the nostrils as foul air. This is performing a revolution of the microcosm, or that which is denoted by *yun-ch'i*. The Taoists prefer retirement to the monasteries in the hills to go through these exercises, as the air there is pure.

功夫 The Dragon Series

The Dragon is the chief among the four divinely constituted beasts, a legendary creature depicted by Chinese tradition as a huge four-footed reptile. The feminine watery principle of the atmosphere is pre-eminently associated with it.

1. The Dragon Stamping the Earth, or The Earth-Stamping Dragon [and so with all the other titles]

Let both hands embrace both shoulders crosswise; fix the toes on the ground, and stamp with the heels 24 times. This is used for strengthening the ligaments and bones. Stamping with the heel causes the blood to circulate in heaven and earth, high and low [that is, all over the body]. The blood and air thus circulating everywhere, boils, abscesses, etc., will not be produced. In this way, people can voluntarily and gratuitously strengthen themselves.[1]

2. The Dragon Wagging His Tail

Place both legs firmly together, and move from side to side like a dragon's tail, 24 times. For pacifying and making comfortable the ligaments and bones. [These results are produced by the movement of the coccyx.]

---

[1]These directions are usually in rhyme, so as to be easily committed to memory. They speak invariably of blood and air; together, these words stand for the constitution. Original air is supposed to be mixed with the blood and to be the cause of its onward movement.

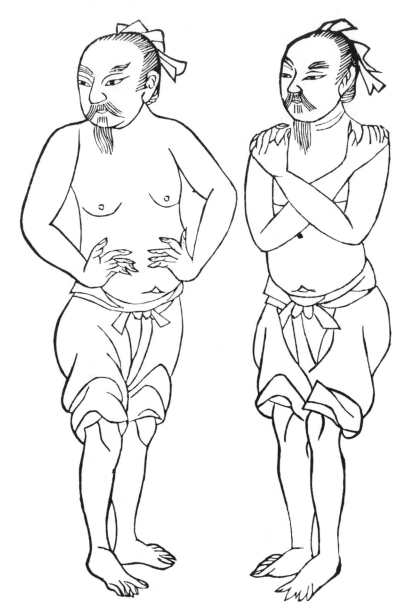

3. The Dragon Rubbing His Head

Take hold of the Dragon with the left hand, and rub his head with the right hand; seize it slowly, and afterwards move it firmly; do not be afraid to repeat it any number of times. The black dragon is the liver, and the white tiger is the lungs. By so manipulating, hardness will disappear, and the dragon will not be afraid at the sight of the tiger.

4. The Whirling-Wind Dragon

With closed fists and head slightly bent downwards, strike out first the right hand and then the left, each hand following the other. This is in order to move the bones and muscles and cause the blood to advance forwards, and so prevent the body from becoming weak.

5. The Dragon Joining His Feet

Sitting straight, place first one leg and then the other in the opposite axilla, and grasp the opposite elbows with the hands. To cause the blood to pass down the vertebrae to the kidneys and coccyx.

6. The Dragon Shutting the Pass

Lift up the hands with the palms towards heaven, thus driving the air up to the head. To be done 24 times; if the air reaches to the *ni-wan* bone,[2] the organs of vision and hearing will be strengthened.

7. The Dragon Closing in the Inspired Air

Maintain perfect quiet, without which the exercise is useless. To be done 81 times. To impart strength.

8. The Dragon Supporting Heaven

The object of this movement is to cause the air to pass from all parts of the body to the coccyx. Lie on the back; the heart is empty [free from all care, etc.], the legs are drawn up, and the hands clasped underneath, 81 times. By this *kung-fu* alone can the air freely circulate to the coccyx.

9. The Ascending Dragon

Sit cross-legged; the breath is retained and drawn into the abdomen, and the mouth is closed and the tongue thrown against the palate. Prescribed for driving out cold, with the hands in the loins, and against incontinence of urine.

Inspire by the nose 90 times. If inspiration by the nose is not attended to, the passages will be blocked up; if the mouth is not closed, the dorsal muscles will be rendered uncomfortable; if the tongue is not

---

[2]"Mud pellet bone," so called from its containing the brain, called the "mud pellet palace," and this again from a reference in the Han dynasty to an official who, with such a pellet, could close the Han Pass.

rubbed against the palate, the air from below will not pass to the occi-put. All pass round like the flowing of the Yellow River and the tides of the ocean and go into the heart.

There are three more given to complete the dozen, forming the Dragon Set: The Dragon Taking Water, The Dragon Fearing Fire, and The Dragon Meditating on the Elixir. These, not being very different from some others already given, are omitted.

功夫 The Tiger Series

The Tiger is the greatest of the four-footed creatures, the lord of wild animals, and represents the masculine principle of nature. His claws act as a talisman; the ashes of his skin, when worn about the person, act as a charm against disease. In Taoist literature, the Dragon and the Tiger play a most important part.

1. The Mountain-Jumping Tiger

Jump from one place to another, and then back, 24 times. In this way, the black dragon and white tiger are brought face to face, and the door of the hill [to become an Immortal] will be opened.

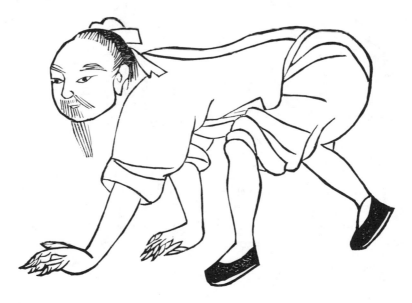

2. The Tiger Coming out of the Cave

On all fours, move backwards and forwards, each 12 times. The muscles and bones are thus made and kept movable, the viscera enjoy peace, and the blood and veins flow regularly.

3. The Flying-Rainbow Tiger

Stretch out the two arms together in one direction, first to the left and then to the right, 24 times, as if flying to the right and the left. This opens the chest and makes it feel comfortable. The muscles, bones, and heart are likewise benefited, and so disease is prevented.

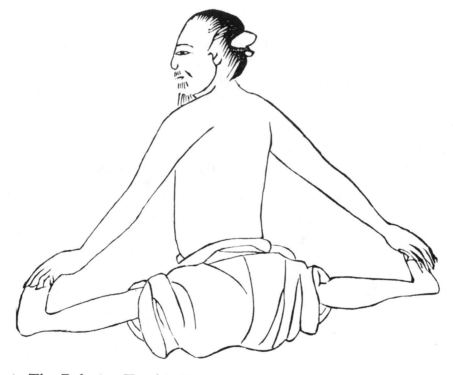

4. The Relaxing-Tendon Tiger

Stretch out both legs flat on the ground, with the arms grasping the feet like the string of a bow, turning to the right and left 12 times each way. With the view of moving the muscles, ligaments and bones, this prevents the production of disease, or removes it far off.

5. The Tiger Suspended from a Beam

Hang the body suspended from a cross-bar, first on one hand, then on the other, 24 times; all manner of diseases will vanish, the air and blood will circulate and the viscera be made comfortable.

6. The Tiger Fixed like the Tripod of an Incense Burner

Sit cross-legged and straight, with hands at the side like a tripod firmly fixed, the shoulders placed straight, and the head thrown up 24 times. This is considered great *kung-fu*, and is calculated to produce great good.

7. The Standing-on-One-Leg Tiger

First on one side, and then on the other, each 12 times. To give peace to the bones and ligaments of the entire body.

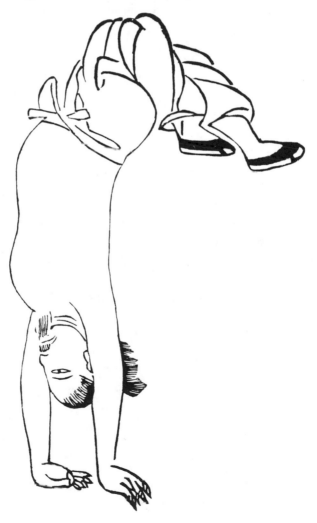

8. The Turning-His-Body Tiger

As if the feet were flying, support the body with the two hands on the ground. To be done 24 times without stopping. To prevent the air stopping anywhere and causing debility and laziness of the body.

9. The Tiger Turning Himself

Turn the hands with palms backwards, and grasp the shoulders firmly 81 times. Used for broadening the chest, and causing the blood and air to move constantly.

10. The Tiger Swallowing Saliva

The saliva is swallowed 24 times. To diminish the fire [inflammation] of the heart.

11. The Peach-Blossom Tiger[1]

Rough the face with both hands. The voice is to be thrown out by pronouncing *ha* until the face is red and quite hot, has no wrinkles, and is as if the person had been drinking.[2]

12. The Peaceful-Spirit Tiger

Sit cross-legged, to pacify the heart, as if looking at a beautiful garden or picture.

13. The Tiger [-woman] Playing the Dragon's Flute

There are no holes in the sides; therefore it is played at the end. If it is not blown, the air cannot enter; if the air does not enter, the road is not open; if the road is not open, the *tan-t'ien* air does not move, and the person is not able to play. If it succeeds, the *tan-t'ien* air passes to the "Heavenly Door," and so round the entire body, according to the diagram illustrative of the *Physiology of Kung-fu.*

14. The Dragon [-man] Playing the Tiger's Guitar

To cause the heart to desire and wish for things, and then both their hearts will be joyful and contract no disease.

---

[1]The peach tree is an ancient symbol of longevity and immortality. It occupies a prominent position in the mystical beliefs of the Taoists, and magical virtues were very early attributed to twigs of this tree.
[2][Ed. note: The Chinese believe that a person of good character will have brightly flushed cheeks when intoxicated.]

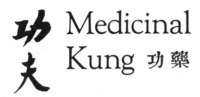 Medicinal Kung 功藥

Experimenting with any exercise without proper guidance can be dangerous. Improperly performed, the exercises may produce no results and can even cause injury or illness. Chinese herbal medicine is not to be taken lightly, and some of the prescriptions may be harmful if taken by the wrong person or at the wrong time. A Chinese doctor or herbalist should be consulted about all matters pertaining to health.

In the following exercises with prescriptions, the Chinese characters with the botanical identification of the substances will be inserted only on their first occurrence. Where the substance is well known, its common and popular name only will be used. [Editor's note: The reader may refer to the Appendix for full listings—romanization, Chinese characters, and botanical identification—for each substance.]

As the illustrations are too numerous and occupy too much space, they are omitted unless the positions or figures are more or less striking; where they resemble or are identical with those already given, reference to the illustration is sufficient.

1. The Honourable and Real Form of the Great Pure Ancestral Teacher

To cure pain in the abdomen and suddenly alternating cold and hot.

In one work this Figure is termed Twisting (or Pressing) and Holding the *Tan-t'ien*: for the cure of abdominal pain and nourishing the strength of the male principle.

The illustration is that of a Taoist priest sitting crosslegged as described.

Sit upright; with both hands embrace below the navel; wait till the *tan-t'ien* is warmed; perform the *kung*, revolving the air in 49 mouthfuls.

THE LEADING AIR SOUP

Prescription Take of *ts'ang-shu* (or *ts'ang-chu*) 苍 术 , Atractylis ovata; *hsiang-fu* 香 附 , Cyperus rotundus; *ch'en-p'i* 陳 皮 , orange peel; *ch'uan-hsiung* 川 芎 , Pleurospermum Sp. or Conioselinum univita-tum (umbelliferae); *pai-chih* 白 芷 , root of Angelica anomala; *fu-ling* 茯 苓 , fungoid growths on roots of Pachyma cocos; *t'u-fu-ling* 土 茯 苓 , root of the smilax (China-root); *shen-ch'u* 神 麯 , a cele-brated medicine cake for curing colds and dispersing wind, brought from Chin-chew near Amoy (the name means "divine leaven"); *tzu-su* 紫 蘇 , Perilla ocymoides; dried ginger; and licorice—of each the same quantity. Make a decoction in water.

2. The Venerable Prince Li Playing the Lute

To cure chronic disease and yellow swelling.

The Figure given in the books is that of the Founder of Taoism. He is popularly termed Lao-Tzu, the Old Child, from the white appearance of his head and the aged appearance of his face at birth. The epithet really means the Old Master. His surname, Li, was derived from the name for the plum tree, under which he was said to have been born. He may have been a contemporary of Confucius. The illustration is, as described, an attitude of meditation assumed by Taoist and Buddhist priests.

Sit silently with both hands on the knees; rub forcibly; let the heart consider and wait till the air has circulated to all parts of the body, and make it go round in 49 mouthfuls. The air will thus revolve, the blood harmonize, and diseases vanish.

THE JUJUBE IRON PILLS

Prescription Take of *lu-fan* 綠 礬 , green alum (sulphate of iron?) burnt; orange peel; and *ts'ang-shu*—of each 2 ounces; *sha-jen* 砂 仁 , cardamoms—3 mace; dried ginger—2 mace; *chih-ch'io*, or *chih-k'o* 枳 殼 , Aegle sepiaria (large fruit); *pin-lang* 檳 榔 , Areca catechu (betel-nut); and *jen-shen* 人 參 , ginseng, root of Aralia quinquefolia (Pansax Ginseng)—of each 3 mace. Powder; boil the jujubes and beat them into a pulp; mix the powder, and make into pills. Dose: 49 morning and evening, to be taken with rice gruel. Fish, fowl, cold and raw articles, and fatty substances are contra-indicated.

After each Prescription, there is a stanza of poetry. The older work consulted omits the poetry. The stanza accompanying this recipe reads:

At first when there was chaos, there was the female principle, then there ascended the male principle, and heaven was divided; the former principle increased, the latter diminished, and then both harmonized; heaven and earth then appeared, and the Great Reason, and this was Creation.

3. Hsu Shen-weng's 徐 神 翁 Method of Preserving the Air and Opening the Passes

To cure false satiety [*i.e.*, being empty and yet having the feeling of fullness].

The closed places, or passes, are:
1. The mouth, the door of the lungs.
2. The teeth, the leaves of the door.
3. The larynx, the inspiratory door. (The sounds in Chinese for expiration and inspiration resemble the sounds produced by the acts, as for example *hu-hsi*, to expire and inspire respectively.)
4. The gullet, the mouth of the stomach.
5. The cardiac orifice.
6. The pyloric orifice.
7. The anus.

The soul goes by the head in the good, and by the fundament in the bad, into the earth. The nine openings of the body do not here require to be specified.

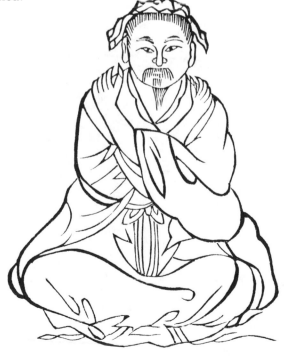

Sit firmly; place the two hands cross-wise on the shoulders [the naked beggars adopt this attitude in winter to keep themselves warm]; let the eyes look to the left side; move the air round in 12 mouthfuls; then turn the eyes to the right, and respire as before.

THE PROTECTING HARMONY PILLS

Prescription Take of *shan-ch'a-jou* 山 查 肉 , fruit of Crataegus pinnatifida—2 ounces; *shen-ch'u* (fried); *pan-hsia* 半 夏 , tubers of Pinellia tuberifera (or rad. Ari macrori); ginger juice to be beaten with it; and *fu-ling*—of each 1 ounce; *lo-fu-tzu* 羅 蔔 子 , Raphanus sativus (radish seeds) (fried); orange peel; *lien-ch'iao* 連 翹 ; and lotus fruit—of each 5 mace. Powder and form the *shen-ch'u* into a paste, with which to make the pills. Dose: 30 to 50, to be taken in a little soup (hot water).

4. The Immortal with the Iron Staff Pointing the Way
For the cure of paralysis.

The Immortal with the Iron Staff is included by Taoist writers in the category of the Eight Immortals. His surname was Li. He is largely represented in Chinese legendary lore, but no precise period is assigned to his existence upon earth. His disembodied spirit entered the body of a

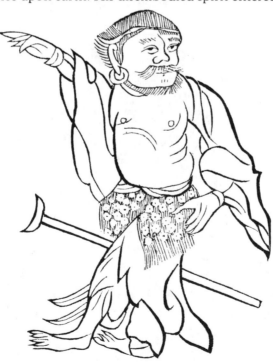

lame and crooked beggar, and in this shape the philosopher continued his existence, supporting his halting footsteps with an iron staff. Hence his name, *T'ieh Kuai*.

Stand firmly, point with the right hand to the right, eyes directed to the left; move the air round in 24 mouthfuls. Let the left foot point to the front; look to the right and left; move the air round in 24 mouthfuls; then put the right foot in front.

THE HARMONIZING AIR POWDER

Prescription Take of *ma-huang* 麻 黃 , Ephedra vulgaris; orange peel; *wu-yao* 烏 藥 , Daphnidium myrrha; *pai-chiang-ts'an* 白 殭 蠶 ; *ch'uan-hsiung*; and *pai-chih*—of each 1 mace; licorice; *chieh-keng* 桔 梗 , Platycordon grandiflorum; and dried ginger—of each 5 candareens; *chih-ch'io*—1 mace. To be taken in boiled water, in which 3 slices of ginger have been digested.

5. The Maiden Immortal Ho 何 仙 姑 Slowly Ascending to Heaven

To cure gravel twisting the intestines and abdominal pain.

In one work, the Figure—a male—is termed The Eighty-one (9 x 9) Ways of Ascending to Heaven.

This maiden is one of the Eight Immortals. When she was born, six hairs were seen growing on the crown of her head. At fourteen she

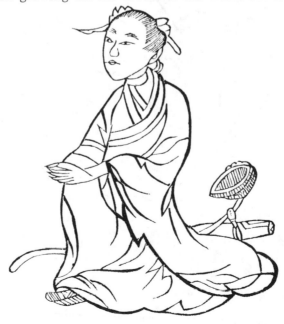

dreamed that a spirit gave her instruction in the art of procuring immortality, for which she was to eat powdered mother-o'-pearl. She
vowed herself to a life of virginity, wandered in the mountains, lived on
herbs, and ultimately disappeared from mortal view. She has since, it is
said, been seen twice.

Sit inclined, the two hands embracing the knees on a level with the
navel; tread up and down with the right and left feet 9 times; move the
air round with 24 mouthfuls.

THE SALT SOUP (WATER) METHOD
FOR BRINGING ON VOMITING

Prescription Use very much salted water to cause vomiting, and the
affection is cured.

6. Pai Yü-ch'an 白 玉 蟾 Seizing His Food Like the Tiger

To cure twisting intestinal gravel.

This Figure is elsewhere termed The Hungry Tiger Seizing His Food.

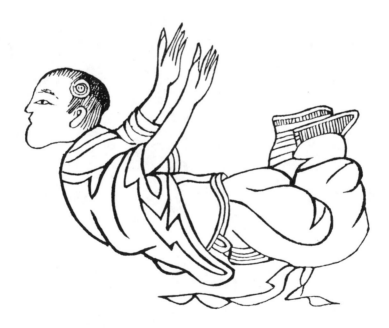

The abdomen to the ground, turn the hands and feet upwards with
force; move the air in 12 mouthfuls; and move the hands and feet right
and left 3 x 5 (15) times. Then firmly sit up erect; make the air advance
by this *kung* in some 14 mouthfuls.

Prescription Take red earth and alum—of each 5 mace. Powder; use one bowl of cold water and mix; allow it to settle, and then drink.

7. Han Chung-li's 漢 鍾 離 Method of Sounding the "Heavenly Drum"

To cure vertigo.

Sometimes called the Vertigo-curing Tiger, or the Peach Blossom Tiger.

A similar exercise is given under the heading, The Hands Beating the Wind Residence [acupuncture aperture below the occipital protuberance] Causing Thunder: for the cure of headache from inflammation of the membranes or from wind.

Bite the teeth, sit straight, shut the breath; use both hands and cover the ears; beat the "Heavenly Drum" 36 times; again tap the teeth 16 times.

ADDING TO THE TASTE OF THE WHITE TIGER SOUP

Prescription Take of gypsum (roasted)—2 candareens; *chih-mu* 知 母 , Anemmorrhena asphodeloides; and licorice—of each 1 mace; *pan-hsia*— 2 candareens; *mai-tung* 麥 冬 , tubers of Ophiopogon japonicus—8 candareens; *chu-yeh* 竹 葉 , bamboo leaves—5 candareens; rice—a picule. Make a decoction with 3 slices of ginger in it. [The heart will thus become as bright as a mirror, and as clear as Heaven—the first couplet of the poetical stanza].

8. The Immortal Maiden Ts'ao 曹 仙 姑 Looking at the Figure of the Ultimate Principle of Being 太 極

To cure inflammation, pain, and swelling of the eyes.
[Ed.: An important practice in Taoist yoga.]

Fix the tongue on the palate; direct the eyes to the vertex and nose (alternately); cause the fire of the heart to descend to and enter the *yung-chuan* (acupuncture aperture in the centre of the sole of the foot); draw up the kidney water (semen) to the *k'un-lun*. In performing it, do it 3 times each time; set it on fire in 36 mouthfuls.

THE BRIGHT EYE FLOWING AIR POTION

Prescription Tang-kuei 當 歸 , Ligusticum acutilobum; *pai-shao* 白 芍 , Paeonia albiflora; *sheng-ti* 生 地 , Rehmannia glutinosa; *lung-tan-ts'ao* 龍 膽 草 , Gentiana scabra; *ch'ai-hu* 柴 胡 , Bupleurum falcatum; *huang-lien* 黃 連 , rhizome of Coptis teeta; *chih-tzu* 梔 子 , Gardenia florida; and *tan-p'i* 丹 皮 , root bark of Paeonia montan—of each 1 mace. Take of rhubarb, boiled in wine, dried and again boiled and dried 3 x 7 (21) times—2 mace; make a decoction and drink.

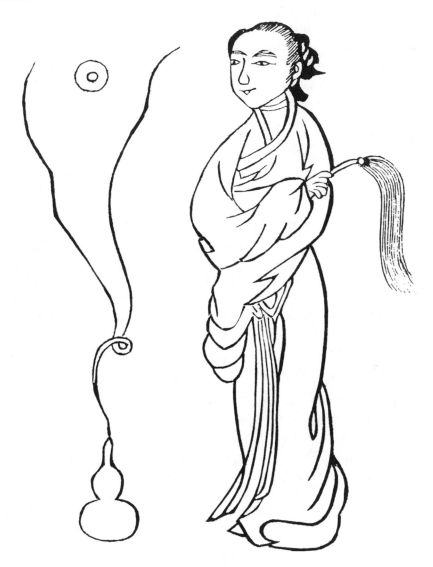

9. Ch'iu Ch'ang-ch'un's 丘 長 春 **Method of Turning the Windlass; otherwise called The Immortal Turning the Windlass [the Shoulder]**

To cure severe pain of the back and arm.

Sit high (as on a chair); extend the right and left feet inclined; press the knees with the two hands, moving the air round in 12 mouthfuls. Do it daily 3 x 5 (15) times.

THE MOVING AIR SOUP

Prescription Take of *kao-pen* 藁 本 , Nothosmyrnium japonicum; *fang-feng* 防 風 , Peucedanum terebinthaceum (?) (root of an umbellifera); and *ch'uan-hsiung*—of each 1 mace; *ch'iang-huo* 羌 活 , Peucedanum decursivum; and *tu-huo* 獨 活 , Angelica inaequalis—of each 2 mace; *man-ching-tzu* 蔓 荊 子 , a kind of turnip with a white tuber below ground—6 candareen; licorice—5 candareens. Boil in water, and drink.

10. Ma Tan-yang's Method of Using the Strength of Fire for the Whole Body 馬 丹 陽 週 天 火 候 訣

To cure the primordial air in a debilitated condition.

Sit firmly cross-legged; first rub the two hands warm, then rub the eyes; afterwards use them to sustain below the ribs on the two sides. When the air advances, rouse it to go upwards, and move the air round in 12 mouthfuls.

THE GINSENG ASTRAGALUS SOUP

Prescription Take of ginseng; *huang-ch'i* 黃 芪, Astragalus; *pai-shu* 白 朮 ; and *tang-kuei*—of each 2 mace; orange peel; *fu-ling*; and licorice—of each 1 mace. Add ginger and jujubes, and boil in water.

11. Chang Tzu-yang 張 紫 陽 Driving the Pestle

To cure indigestion, or distension and rumbling of the abdomen, with pain each time.

Stand firmly; support heaven with the two hands; stamp the earth, and circulate the air 9 times.

THE SOUP FOR WIDENING THE CENTRE [THORAX]

Prescription Take of *tzu-su; keng-yeh* 梗 葉, Hemiptelea Davidi (Zelkora Davidi); cardamons; *chih-ch'io; ch'ing-p'i* 青 皮 , immature fruits (dried) of a species of citrus; orange peel; betel-nut; *mu-hsiang* 木 香 , root of Aplotaxis auriculata (putchuck); *pan-hsia; lo-fu-tzu; hou-p'o* 厚 朴 , flowers of the Szechuan *hou-p'o-tzu; ts'ang-shu; tse-hsieh* 澤 瀉 , Alisma plantago; and *mu-t'ung* 木 通 , Clematis—of each the same; crude ginger—2 slices boiled in water.

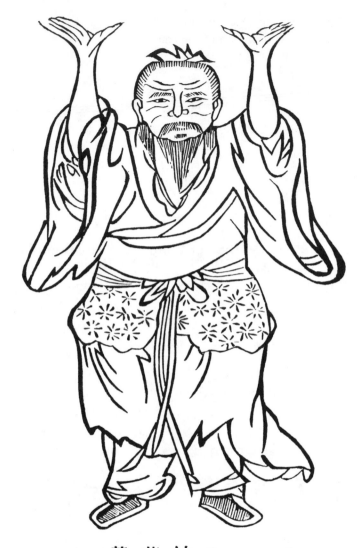

12. Miss Huang-hua 黄 花 姑 Sleeping on Ice

To cure consumption and extreme debility from venereal excesses.

Lie with the left hand for a pillow; rub the abdomen with the right fist; flex the right foot a little; press the right leg upon the left a little; as if sleeping in this manner, inspire 32 mouthfuls, and move the air round in 12 mouthfuls.

THE SOUP OF THE GREAT SHOP
FOR STRENGTHENING THE CENTRE [THORAX]

Prescription Take of ginseng; *pai-shu*; *fu-ling*; *pai-shao*; *shu-ti* 熟 地

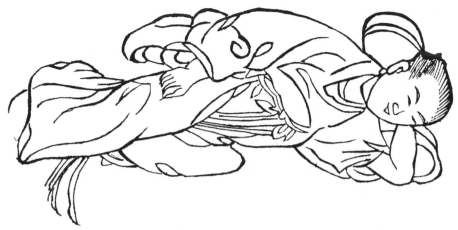

(see *sheng-ti*); and *huang-ch'i*—of each 1 mace; *tang-kuei*; *ch'uan-hsiung*; *tu-chung* 杜 仲 , bark of an Euphorbiaceous tree; *ts'ung-jung* 從 蓉 , Aeginetia Sp.; and *ku-chih* 故 紙 , legumes of Psoralea (Bauchee seeds) —of each 7 candareens; licorice; and cinnamon—of each 3 candareens. Boil with ginger and jujubes, and take at any time.

13. Yin Ch'ing-ho's 尹 清 和 Sleeping Plan

To cure weakness of the spleen and stomach, and indigestion of the five cereals [hemp-seed, millet, rice, wheat and pulse].

Recline on the back; place the right foot like a frame on the left foot; lay the two hands straight on the shoulders, the abdomen coming and going; move the air round in 6 mouthfuls.

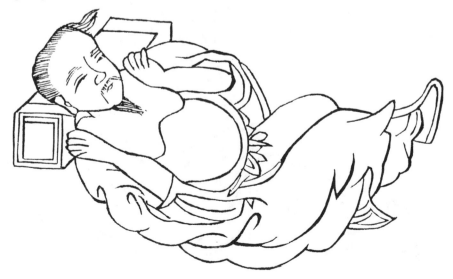

THE STRONG SPLEEN PILLS

Prescription Take of *pai-shu* (roasted with earth); *chih-shih* 枳實 (roasted), Aegle sepiaria (small fruit); orange peel; *mai-ya* 麥芽 (roasted), sprouts of wheat and barley; *shen-ch'u* (roasted); *shan-yao* 山 藥, Dioscorea Sp. (yams); *fu-ling*; and *ts'ang-shu* (roasted)—of each 1 ounce; *hou-p'o* (prepared)—8 mace; *mu-hsiang*—5 mace. Powder; take non-glutinous rice flour, make into a paste, and form pills. Dose: 6 or 7 in rice gruel.

14. Li Ch'i-ch'an's 李 棲 蟾 Method of Dispersing the Semen (Ching 精)

Sometimes called Lu-tsu's Method for Strengthening the Semen: to cure spermatorrhea from dreams.

Sit upright; raise up both feet and rub the soles until warm; move the air right and left each in 30 mouthfuls; and so the semen will not flow away. [The Chinese believe that the *ching* is secreted in the kidneys and can be dispersed throughout the entire body, thus preventing it from collecting and flowing away.]

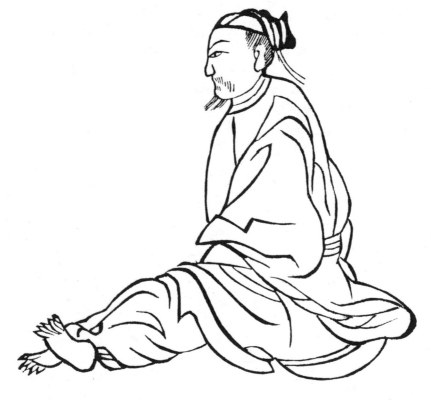

THE STRONG CHING PILLS

Prescription Take of *chih-mu* (roasted); and *huang-po* 黃 栢, Phelloden-dron amurense or Pterocarpus flavus—of each 1 ounce; burnt oyster shells; burnt fossil bones; *tz'u-shih* 芡 實, Euryale ferox; *lien-jui*, stamens of lotus flowers; *fu-ling*; *yuan-chih* 遠 志, root and root bark of Polygala sibirica; and *shan-chu-yü* 山 茱 萸, fruit of a shrub not yet identified—of each 2 ounces. Powder boiled rice and make the pills with a cinnabar coating. Dose: 50 pills on an empty heart [stomach]; swallow with diluted salted water.

15. The Maiden Chang Chen-nu 張 眞 奴 Fixing Her Animal Spirits

To cure emptiness and great pain of the heart.

Sit upright; press the knees with the two hands; use the idea in it; look to the right and elevate the left; move the air in 12 mouthfuls; look to the left and raise the right; and move the air in 12 mouthfuls.

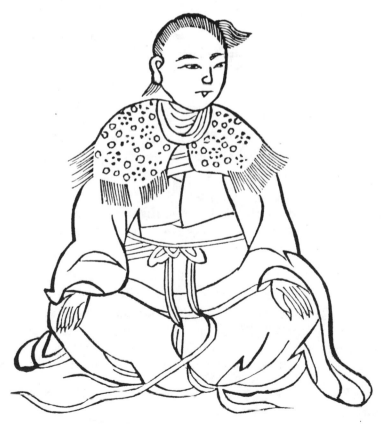

THE PAIN-REMOVING POWDER

Prescription Take of *wu-ling-chih* 五 靈 脂 , magpie's dung; *p'u-huang* 蒲 黃 , Typha sp. (roasted); and *tang-kuei*—of each 1 ounce; *mou-kuei*, Cinnamomum cassia; *mu-hsiang*; and *shih-ch'ang-p'u* 石菖蒲 , Acorus gramineus—of each 8 mace. Powder and boil. Dose: 4 mace, to be boiled with a little salt and vinegar.

16. Wei Po-yang's 魏 伯 陽 Method of Beating the Wind
To cure chronic paralysis.

Wei Po-yang was a celebrated Taoist philosopher and alchemist of the Han dynasty, who is known to have devoted himself to the preparation of the elixer of immortality, and who is the author of a professed commentary on the *I Ching* (Book of Changes).

Sit upright; place the right fist against the right ribs; press the knee with the left hand; extend and withdraw the feet; think; move the air to the diseased part, right and left, each in 6 mouthfuls.

THE GOLD-PRODUCING TIGER-BONES POWDER

Prescription Take of *tang-kuei*; *ch'ih-shao* 赤 芍 , Paeonia albiflora (the cultivated variety which bears red flowers); *ch'uan-hsu-tuan* 川 續 斷 , Dipsacus asper or Lamium album from Szechuan; *pai-shu*; *kao-pen*; and tigers' bones—of each 1 ounce; *shao-wu-she-jou* 稍 烏 蛇 肉—5 mace. Powder. Dose: 2 mace, to be swallowed with tepid wine.

17. Hsueh Tao-kuang 薛 道 光 Rubbing His Heel
For nourishing the original essence.

The Figure resembles number 8 of the Ornamental Sections, and is therefore omitted.

Sit straight; rub with the hands until the sole of the left foot is warm; move the air in 24 mouthfuls; afterwards rub the sole of the right foot warm, the rest the same as the left.

THE EXTRACT OF TWO IMMORTALS, KUEI AND LU
[THE TORTOISE AND THE DEER]

Prescription Take of deer horns—10 catties; shell of a land tortoise—5 catties; *kou-ch'i-tzu* 枸 杞 子 , Lycium chinense—30 ounces; and ginseng—15 ounces. Use a jar and make it after the manner of an extract; then dissolve it in wine. Dose: 2 to 3 or 4 mace on an empty stomach.

18. Ko Hsien-weng 葛 僊 翁 Opening the Thorax
To cure the thorax of obstruction.

Stand erect, the feet placed after the Chinese character for "8" 八 ; interlock the two hands and carry them to the front of the chest; rub them times without number, and move the air in 34 mouthfuls.

Another plan is to direct the left hand, using force, to the left, the right hand also forcibly following the left; direct the head also with strength to the right, the eyes strongly directed to the right; move the air in 9 mouthfuls; change the hands and repeat.

THE POWDER FOR WIDENING THE CENTRE

Prescription Take of *chih-ch'io* (roasted); *chieh-keng*; *fu-ling*; *pan-hsia*; orange peel; *hou-p'o, hsiang-fu*; and *sha-jen*—of each the same quantity. Add a few slices of ginger, and make a decoction.

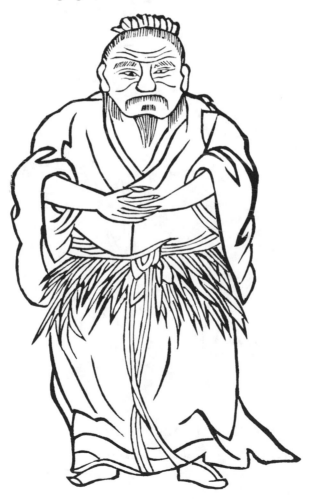

19. Wang Yü-yang's 王 玉 陽 Method of Dispersing Pain

To cure periodical air and a painful condition of the whole body.

Stand upright firmly; let the left foot be carried to the front and the right to the back; place the two fists on the belly; move the air in 24 mouthfuls. The exercise is the same on the right and left.

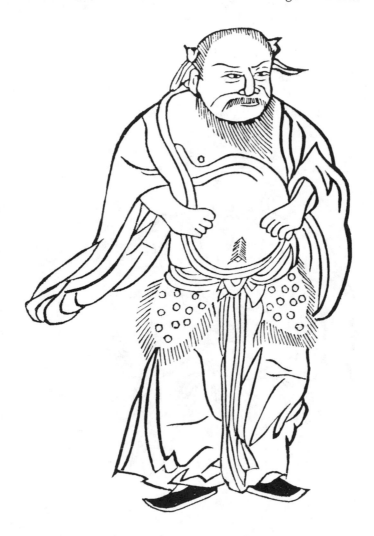

THE GINSENG HARMONIZING AIR POWDER

Prescription Take of *ch'uan-hsiung; chieh-keng; pai-chih;* orange peel; *chih-ch'io;* licorice; *ma-huang; wu-yao;* ginseng; and *ch'iang-huo*—of each 7 candareens. Make a decoction.

20. The Maiden Ma 麻 姑 Rubbing [away] the Disease
To cure imperviousness of the air and arteries.

Ma Ku (Maiden Ma) is one of the female celebrities of Taoist fable, a sister of the immortalized soothsayer and astrologer Wang Yuan of the Han dynasty.

Except that the hand is pointing, this Figure of Miss Ma resembles that of Miss Ts'ao (number 8), who is viewing the Absolute, from which is evolved the two primordial essences, or male and female principles.

Stand firmly. If it is the air and blood vessels of the left side that are not pervious [*i.e.*, not circulating so as to reach all points], then the right hand acts the *kung*, and the idea or thought is to be directed to the left. If it is the right side that is impervious, the left hand acts, and the will is to be on the right. Each side is to have 5 mouthfuls of the revolving air.

THE PUTCHUCK FLOWING AIR POTION

Prescription Take of *pan-hsia*; *ch'ing-p'i*; licorice; *o-shu* 莪 术 , Kampferia pandurata; betel-nut; *hsiang-fu*; *ts'ao-kuo* 草 菓 , Amomus medium (Ovoid Chinese cardamon); *pai-chih*; *mu-kua* 木 瓜 , Pyrus Cathayensis (Chinese quince); ginseng; *ch'ih-fu-ling*; red variety *mu-t'ung*; *huo-hsiang* 藿 香 , Lophantus rugosus (bishopwort); *ting-hsiang*, cloves (flower buds of Eugenia carophyllata); orange peel; *tzu-su, mou-kuei; hou-p'o; mu-hsiang; mai-tung; pai-shu; ch'ang-p'u*, Acorus calamus; and *ta-fu* 大 腹 , betel-nut skin. Add 3 slices of ginger and 1 jujube, and make a decoction.

21. The Picture of Chang Kuo-lao Abstracting from and Adding to the Strength of Fire 抽 添 火 候
To cure the heat of the blood of the Three Divisions [imaginary functional passages] advancing upwards, and indistinct vision.

The illustration is similar to numbers 2, 9, 10, and 16.

Sit upright; let the hands rub the navel warm; afterwards press the knees, shut the mouth, sit quiet and wait till the air is fixed, then revolve the air in 9 mouthfuls.

THE CHRYSANTHEMUM POWDER

Prescription Take of *ch'iang-huo*; *mu-tsei* 木 賊 , Equisetum japonicum; *huang-lien; ch'uan-hsiung; ching-chieh* 荆 芥 , Salvia plebeia; *fang-feng; tang-kuei; pai-shao*; licorice; *kan-chu-hua* 甘 菊 花 , Chrysanthemum sinense (sweet), a kind exported from Canton; *man-ching-tzu*; and *huang-ch'in* 黄 芩 , Scutellaria viscidula—of each the same. Make a decoction to be taken after food.

22. Ch'en's *Kung* for Obtaining His Great Sleep
To cure cold caught at any of the Four Seasons

One of the most frequently occurring names in the works on Kung-fu is Ch'en Hsi-i, or -t'uan 陳希夷。搏 (died c. 990 A.D.), who seems to have designed many of the Figures for the cure or prevention of disease. The Year's Kung-fu is attributed to him. He was a celebrated Taoist philosopher and recluse who devoted himself to the study of the arts of sublimation and the occult philosophy of the *I Ching*.

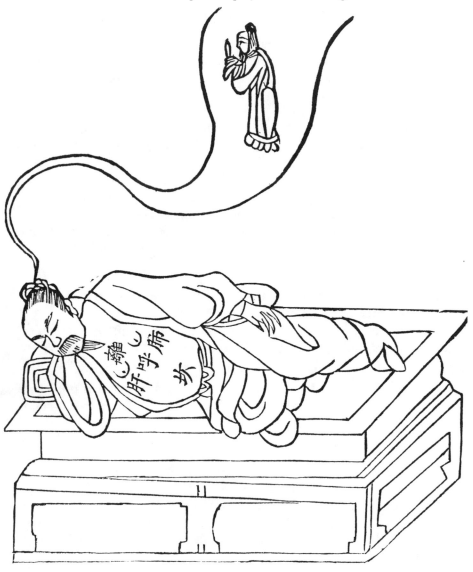

There are illustrations of Ch'en sleeping on the left and right sides in two of the works consulted. They are accompanied by two poetical stanzas, the last line of the left sleeping kung running thus:

"When the tiger and the dragon are collected together at two of the Earthly Branches [related to fire and water], the Great Elixir is complete."

The tiger is here placed on the right, the dragon on the left. In the sleeping exercise for the right side (see illustration), the liver occupies the right and the lungs the left side, with two of the Eight Diagram figures, Li and K'an (fire and water respectively), above and below, and Hu in the middle. The whole stanza reads:

"The air of the lungs resides in the place of the K'an; and liver is directed towards the Li place. Revolve the air [an older work gives spleen air instead] and call it to harmonize in the middle position; the five airs [the atmospheric influences or natures of the Five Elements] collect together as one, and enter the Great Void."

Lie on one side; flex the legs; rub the two hands until warm; embrace the membrum virile and scrotum, and revolve the air in 24 mouthfuls.

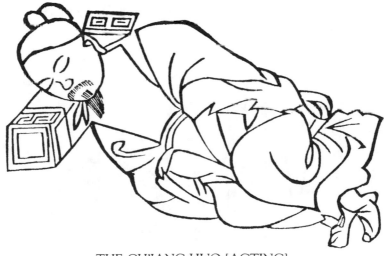

THE CH'IANG-HUO [ACTING]
LIKE A DIVINE POWDER

Prescription Take of *ch'iang-huo; tu-huo; pai-chih;* orange peel; *tzu-su; shan-cha; ts'ao-kuo; fang-feng; kan-ko* 乾 葛 , Pachyrhizus angulatus; *pan-hsia;* licorice; *ts'ang-shu; ch'ai-hu; huang-ch'in;* and *ch'uan-hsiung*—of each 8 candareens; ginger—3 slices; and 3 onion tubers. Make a decoction, and take it hot to produce perspiration.

23. Shih Hsing-lin's 石 杏 林 Method of Warming the Tan-t'ien

To cure the small bowels of air, cold and pain.

The Figure is the usual one, with the hands embracing the navel as directed.

Sit upright; rub the two hands until extremely hot; direct them to the navel, and circulate the air in 49 mouthfuls.

ADDING TO THE TASTE OF THE SAN-LING 三 苓 POWDER

Prescription Take of *chu-ling* 猪 苓 , tuberiform bodies of an unknown nature; *tse-hsieh*; *pai-shu*; cinnamon; *hui-hsiang* 茴 香 , Foeniculum vulgaris (fennel); betel-nut; *mu-t'ung*; *chin-ling-tzu* 金 鈴 子 ; and *chu-ho-jen* 橘 核 仁 , orange seed kernels. Make a decoction, adding a little salt.

24. Han Hsiang-tzu's 韓 湘 子 Figure for Nourishing the Human Heart 活 人 心 .

To cure curvature of the lumbar spine and shaking (palsy) of the head.

In one work the Figure is designated The Dragon Wagging His Tail: for the cure of lumbago.

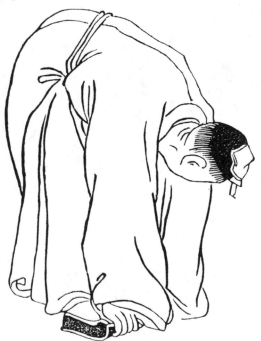

Han Hsiang-tzu was one of the Eight Immortals of Taoist fable, and an ardent votary of transcendental study. A pupil of the patriarch Lu, he was carried up to the famous peach tree and fell from its branches; in descending, he entered upon the state of immortality.

Stand firmly; bend the head; curve the lumbar spine, and perform the act of showing reverence. In doing this *kung*, let the hands and soles of the feet be on the same level. Revolve the air in 24 mouthfuls.

SOUP FOR EXPANDING THE SMALL BLOOD VESSELS

Prescription Take of *ch'iang-huo*; *fang-chi* 防 巳 , roots and bulbs (?); *pai-shu*; *tang-kuei*; *pai-shao*; and *chiang-huang* 姜 黄 , Curcuma longa (turmeric)—of each 1 ounce; licorice—7 mace; *hai-t'ung-p'i* 海 桐 皮 , either Acanthopanax ricinifolium or Bombax malabaricum—1 ounce. Dose: 3 mace, with 10 slices of ginger. Make a decoction.

25. Miss Chao-ling's 昭 靈 女 Manner of Making Disease Go

To cure cold, numbness, and extreme pain of the leg and foot.

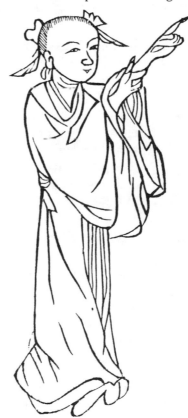

Stand erect; extend a finger of the left hand; with the right hand nip the belly of the arm. Revolve the air in 24 mouthfuls.

A similar exercise is termed The Patriarch Lu's Method of Causing the Blood and Air to Circulate: for the cure of pain of the back and shoulder.

Stretch out the left arm and press the inner aspect of the forearm with the right hand, and *vice versa*. Take 22 breaths.

THE FANG-FENG T'IEN-MA POWDER

Prescription Take of *t'ien-ma* 天 麻 , Gastrodia elata; *fang-feng*; licorice; *ch'uan-hsiung*; *ch'iang-huo*; *tang-kuei*; *pai-chih*; and *hua-shih* 滑 石 , talc—of each 2 ounces; *ts'ao-wu-t'ou* 草 烏 頭 , Aconite; *pai-fu-tzu* 白 附 子 , Arisaema sp.; and *ching-chieh-sui* 荊 芥 穗 —of each 5 mace. Powder; take warm wine and dissolve in a little honey, take ½ to 1 mace; and mix with it. Take of this medicine until you feel slightly numb, and then stop.

26. Lu Ch'un-yang's Figure of Sustaining the Pulse
To cure the hundred [all] diseases.

A similar exercise is elsewhere termed The March of the Blood Vessels.

The Figure resembles number 7 in every respect, and also number 1 of the Ornamental Sections.

Lu Tsu 呂 祖 , or Yen 嵒 , or Tung-pin 洞 賓 , or Ch'un-yang 純 陽 —for he is known by all these names—was born in 755 A.D. He was one of the most prominent of the later patriarchs of the Taoist sect. He was invested with magic formulas and a sword of supernatural powers, with which he traversed the Empire, slaying dragons and ridding the earth of divers kinds of evils during a period of upwards of four hundred years. In the 12th century, temples were erected to his honour and dedicated to his worship under the title Ch'un-yang, which he had adopted. He is worshipped especially by the fraternity of doctors and barbers.

Sit upright; let the two hands press the "sun" and "moon" [two lateral acupuncture apertures two inches below the heart] 9 times; circulate the air 9 mouthfuls.

Another method is to press the knees with the two hands, twist the body right and left, and with each turn of the body revolve the air in 14 mouthfuls.

Prescription Use 1 *wei-ling-hsien* 威 靈 仙, Clematis sp., on the two days known as *ping-ting* 丙 丁 and *hsu-ssu* 戌 巳 , 2 made for a dose in warm wine; avoid tea. To be taken on an empty heart [stomach], and in summer there will be no epidemics, and in autumn no ague and dysentery, and all diseases will be banished easily and without trouble, as the title of the Prescription intimates.

27. Ch'en Hsi-i Imitating the Cow Descending from Looking at the Moon 降牛望月

To cure spermatorrhea only.

This *kung* is sometimes termed A Cow Grasping the Moon.

When there is about to be an emission, let the middle finger of the left hand plug the right nostril, and let the right hand middle finger press the *wei-lu* 尾 閭 aperture [coccyx, where the seminal road or vessel is supposed to be situated], and so stop the flow of the semen; revolve the air in 6 mouthfuls.

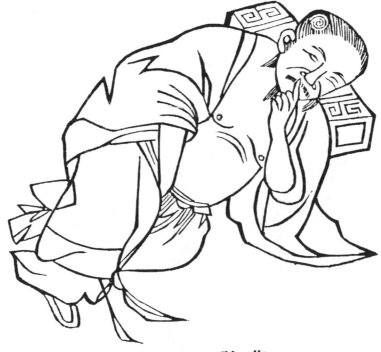

THE SHEN-HSIUNG 神 芎 SOUP

Prescription Take of ginseng; *kou-ch'i-tzu*; *yuan-chih*; *huang-ch'i*; licorice; *kuei-shen* 歸 身 (see *tang-kuei*); *tu-chung* (roasted); *pai-shu*; *ti-ku-p'i* 地 骨 皮 , root bark of Lycium chinense; and *pu-ku-chih* (roasted)—of each the same quantity. Add 1 slice of ginger and 7 lotus seeds deprived of their core. Make a decoction with water, and take.

28. Fu-yu Ti-chun 孚佑帝君 Drawing the Sword from its Scabbard

To cure all sorts of cardiac pains.

This is elsewhere termed The Immortals Unsheathing the Sword: for the cure of cardialgia.

Stand erect and firm like the character 丁 (a nail); raise the right hand and look to the left; if the left hand is raised, look to the right. Revolve the air in 9 mouthfuls, turn the head, and look to the four quarters.

THE FALLING CUP SOUP

Prescription Take of *hsuan-hu-so* 玄 胡 索 , tubers of Corydalis ambigua; *wu-ling-chih* (thoroughly roasted); *chien-k'ou-jen* 建 蔻 仁 , nutmeg kernels from Fukien—of each 6 candareens; *liang-chiang* 艮 薑 , Galangal (alpinia officinarum); *shih-ch'ang-p'u*; *hou-p'o*; orange peel; and *huo-hsiang*—of each 1 mace; *chih-ch'io*; and *su-keng* 蘇 梗 , Perilla ocymoides—of each 6 candareens. Make a decoction with water, and drink.

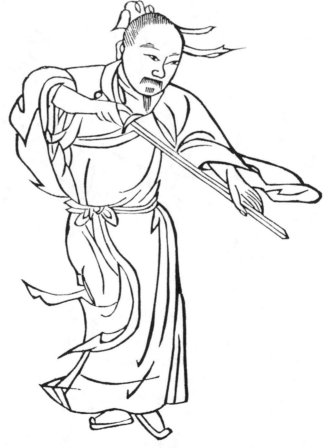

29. The Divine Ancestor Hsu 徐 神 祖 Shaking the "Heavenly Pillar"

To cure all sorts of ulcers on the head, face, shoulders and back.

The Figure resembles numbers 1, 18 (standing), and 23.

Sit upright; let the two hands seize each other below the heart; agitate the "heavenly pillar" right and left; each time, revolve the air, *hem* and blow 24 mouthfuls.

THE POWDER FOR DISPERSING POISON

Prescription Take of *huang-ch'in*; *huang-lien*; rhubarb; *pai-chih*; *ch'iang-huo*; *fang-feng*; *chin-yin-hua* 金 銀 花 , Lonicera japonica; *lien-ch'iao*, values of the fruit of Forsythia suspensa; *tang-kuei*; *ching-chieh*; *t'ien-hua-fen* 天 花 粉 , root of Trichosanthes multiloba; and licorice—equal quantities of each. Make a decoction, and drink.

30. Ch'en Ni-wan's Method of Grasping the Wind's Nest [acupuncture aperture below the occiput; see number 7]

To cure lack of clearness of the brain, and rheumatism of the head. Sit with the back to the outside, and let the two hands embrace the ears and the back of the head. Revolve the air in 12 mouthfuls, and bring the palms together 12 times.

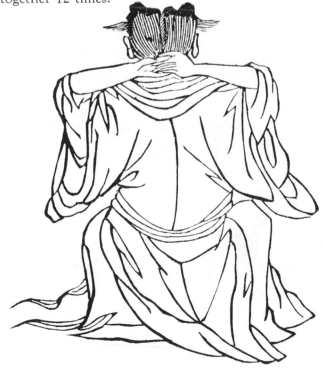

THE CH'IANG-HUO PAI-CHIH SOUP

Prescription Take of *ch'ai-hu*; *fu-ling*; *fang-feng*; *ching-chieh*; *huang-lien*; *tse-hsieh*; *tang-kuei*; *pai-shu*; *man-ching-tzu*; gypsum, *ts'ang-shu*; *hsin-i* 辛 夷 , buds of Magnolia conspicua (or M. Kobus); *sheng-ti*; *ch'uan-hsiung*; *kao-pen*; licorice; *pai-chih*; *ch'iang-huo*; *huang-ch'in*; *hsi-hsin* 細 辛 , Asarum Sieboldi; and *shao-yao* (same as *pai-shao*)—of each the same quantity. Add crude ginger, and make a decoction.

31. Ts'ao Kuo-chiu 曹 國 舅 Taking Off His Boots
To cure pain of the foot, calf, and abdomen.

This exercise is elsewhere called The Immortals Taking Off Their Shoes: for the cure of lumbago.

Ts'ao kuo-chiu was one of the Eight Immortals of Taoist fable.

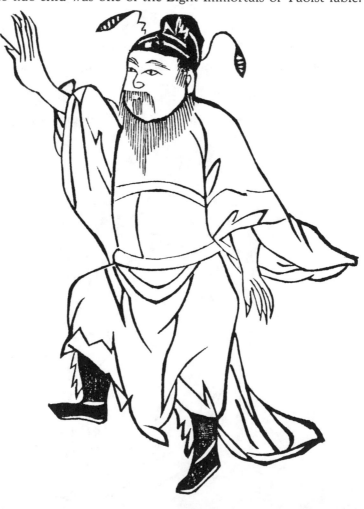

Stand firmly; place the right hand as if scaling a wall and let the left hand hang down; direct the right foot in front and step *in vacuo*. Revolve the air 16 times. The left and right are the same.

THE CH'IANG-HUO SOUP
FOR NOURISHING THE EXHAUSTED

Prescription Take of *ch'iang-huo*; *ch'uan-hsiung*; *ts'ang-shu*; *pai-chih*; *nan-hsing* 南 星 Arisaema japonicum (?); *tang-kuei*; and *shen-ch'u*—of each 1 mace; *sha-jen*; *kuei-chih*, bark of cassia twigs; *fang-chi*; and *mu-t'ung*—of each 8 candareens. Add 3 slices of ginger, and make a decoction.

32. Chao Shang-tsao's 趙 上 灶 Method of Transferring and Stopping the *Ching*

To cure wet dreams.

Sit on one side; use the pair of hands to take hold of the soles of the two feet; first take hold of the left sole and rub it warm, and revolve the air 9 times. Afterwards do the sme with the right sole, and perform the *kung* like the left.

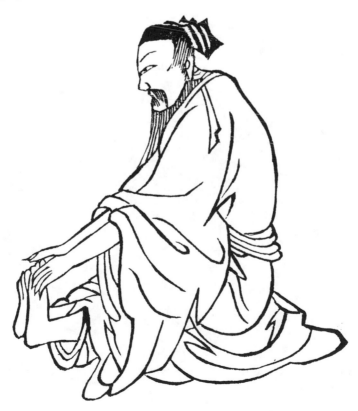

THE JADE PASS PILLS 玉 關 ; YÜ-MEN 玉 門 , THE JADE DOOR, THE CHING DOOR

Prescription Take of ginseng—6 mace; jujube kernels; roasted oyster shells; *wu-pei-tzu* 梧 倍 子 , nut-galls of Rhus semialata (commercial); punjabenis (medicinal); roasted alum; and fossil bones—of each 5 mace; *fu-shen* 伏 神 roots and bulbs—1 ounce; and *yuan-chih* (core to be extracted)—1½ ounces. Steam the jujube kernels, and make the whole into pills. Dose: 50 to 60 on an empty stomach, to be taken in soup made from the seeds of the lotus.

33. The Pure Peaceful Heavenly Preceptor's Sleeping *Kung*

To cure spermatorrhea from dreams.

Recline obliquely on a pillow, with the right hand under the head; with the left rub the abdomen, draw up the legs, the left not quite up to the level of the right and the left pressing on the right; breathe gently, vacant in thought, and take into the abdomen 32 mouthfuls. Do this 12 times. If the exercise is long continued, the disease is certain to be cured.

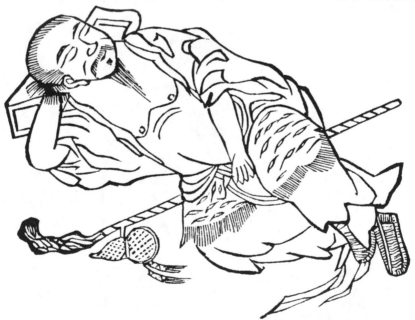

Another similar exercise is simply termed The Sleeping Method: for the cure of nocturnal emissions.

Lie on the back and make a pillow of the right hand; with the left hand press on the thigh of the extended left leg; draw up the right leg, think, and inspire 24 mouthfuls.

There is yet another Sleeping Method: for the cure of dyspepsia.

With both hands rub up and down the abdomen in all directions, like the whirling of a river or the eddying of the ocean.

The above is elsewhere termed The Sleeping Exercise of Ch'en T'uan: for the cure of consumption and the effects of venery.

Recline on the back, the right hand supporting the head [as a pillow], the left hand firmly grasping the obscure parts [the genitals]; extend the left leg straight; flex the right leg; let the heart think and revolve the air 24 times.

THE NOURISHING-HEART SOUP

Prescription Take of ginseng; *shan-yao*; *mu-t'ung*; *fu-shen*; *suan-tsao-jen* 酸 棗 仁 , seeds of Diospyros lotus; *kuei-shen*; clarified *tang-kuei*; *pai-shao*; *yuan-chih* flesh (pulp); and *lien-hsu* 蓮 鬚 (same as *lien-jui*)—of each the same quantity. Add ginger, jujube, and lotus pulp. Make a decoction, and take.

34. Sun Hsuan-hsu 孫 玄 虛 Imitating the Black Dragon Taking Hold of His Claws

To cure pain of the loins and legs.

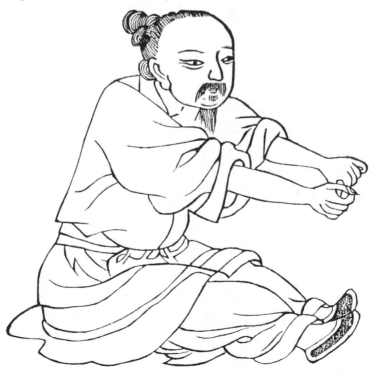

Sit firmly on the ground; extend both feet; push the two hands out in front, and take hold of the two feet on the same level, and come and go, in this way performing the exercise. Revolve the air in 19 mouthfuls.

Elsewhere this exercise appears as The Dragon Grasping His Claws: for the cure of pain of the whole body.

Sit with the body straight, both feet extended together; close and open the fists alternately; stretch the body forward along with the fists, and take 12 mouthfuls.

Another is termed The Tiger Stretching His Claws: for the cure of pain in the back and limbs.

Sit upright with both legs crossed; stretch both arms to the front on a level with the feet; move them backwards and forwards in this manner, so that the air may follow the motions of the arms and thus be introduced into the parts affected.

THE NIU-HSI WINE

Prescription Take of *ti-ku-p'i*; *wu-chia-p'i* 五 加 皮 , Eleutherocrocus; *i-i-jen* 薏 苡 仁 , seeds of Coix lachryma (roasted); *ch'uan-hsiung*; *niu-hsi*—of each 2 ounces; licorice; and *sheng-ti*—3 ounces; *hai-t'ung-p'i*—1½ ounces; *ch'iang-huo*—1 ounce; *tu-chung* (roasted)—2 ounces. Use good wine without lees, to be well digested. Dose: 1 or 2 cupfuls, 3 or 4 times daily, to be drunk before the flavour of the wine has passed off.

35. Kao Hsiang-hsien's 高 象 先 Imitation of the Phoenix Spreading its Wings

To cure diseases the same as the preceding one.

What is translated "phoenix" is a fabulous bird. The male is termed *feng* and the female *huang*; combined they form the bird's generic designation, *feng-huang*. (See illustration in the Year's Kung-Fu)

Bend and contract the body a little; raise the hand higher than the vertex; let the mouth and nose slowly emit the pure air (!) in 3 or 4 mouthfuls; let the left foot be directed to the front, let the toes of the right foot be opposed to the left heel; and revolve the air 10 times.

THE FLOWING AIR POTION

Prescription Take of *ch'-iang-huo*; *ts'ang-shu*; *ch'uan-hsiung*; *tang-kuei*; *hsiang-fu*; *pai-shao*; orange peel; *pan-hsia*; *mu-hsiang*; *chih-ch'io*; *mu-t'ung*; licorice; betel-nut; *tzu-su*—of each the same quantity. Make a decoction.

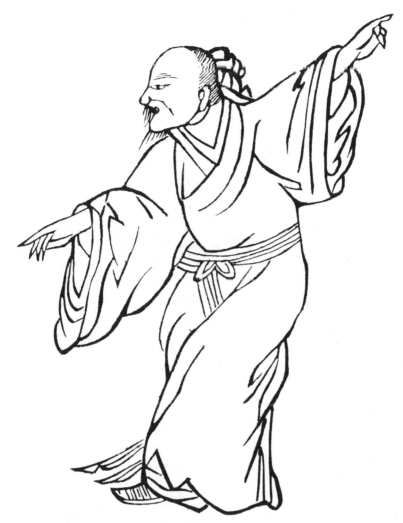

36. Fu Yuan-hsu 傅 元 虚 Embracing the Vertex
To cure vertigo.

Sit upright; rub the two hands warm and embrace the vertex door [anterior fantanelle]; shut the eyes to prevent the animal spirits from being dissipated; blow, *hem*, and drum the air to cause it to ascend to the top of the vertex; revolve the air 17 times.

THE RHUBARB SOUP

Prescription Take of the best rhubarb, and digest it in wine 7 times; dry, and then powder. Use tea. Dose: 3 mace.

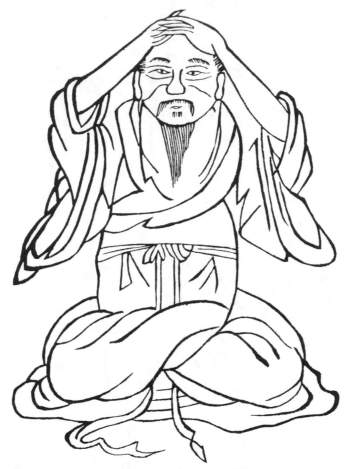

37. The Immortal Li Hung-chi 李 弘 濟 Admiring the Moon
To harmonize the air and invigorate the blood.

Bend the arms as if prostrating oneself to do obeisance; cross the hands and feet; crawl along on the ground; practise the *kung* right and left, and revolve the air each in 12 mouthfuls.

HARMONIZING THE AIR AND NOURISHING
THE BLOOD SOUP

Prescription Take of *tzu-su* (leaves of a stem)—1 mace; *ch'iang-huo*—1 mace; *pan-hsia*; *sang-pai-p'i* 桑 白 皮, root bark of the mulberry (Morus alba); *ch'ing-p'i*; orange peel; and *ta-fu-p'i* 大 腹 皮, same as betel-nut—of each 8 candareens; *ch'ih-fu-ling*; and *mu-t'ung*—of each 8 candareens; *ch'ih-shao*—1 mace; licorice—5 candareens; *tang-kuei*—1 mace; and *mou-kuei*—3 candareens. Make a decoction.

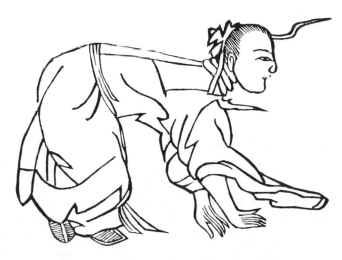

38. Li T'ieh-kuai the Immortal Leaning on His Staff
To cure pains of the loins and back.

Place the hands to the back and stand firm; take the staff to buttress the loins; let the left side lean on the staff; revolve the air 108 times; divide

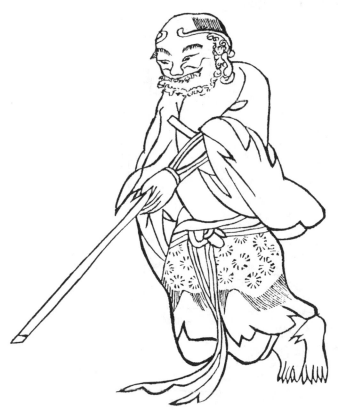

into 3 mouthfuls and swallow; afterwards kneel, and swing from side to side as if sweeping the ground. Do it on the right side in like manner.

This Figure is elsewhere called the Immortal Leaning on a Stick: for the cure of lumbago.

Take 18 mouthfuls 3 times, and move the legs alternately, as if sweeping the floor.

THE TANG-KUEI METHOD OF PICKING OUT PAIN

Prescription Take of *ch'iang-huo*; licorice, *huang-ch'in* (digested in wine); *yin-ch'en* 茵 陳 , Artemisia sp. (roasted in wine)—of each 5 mace; *k'u-shen* 苦 參 , root of Sophora flavescens or gustifolia; *ko-ken* 葛 根 , Pachyrhisus angulatus; and *ts'ang-shu*—of each 2 mace; *fang-feng*; *kuei-shen* (clarified); *chih-mu* (washed in wine); ginseng; *sheng-ma* 升 麻 , Astilbe chinensis; *fu-ling*; *tse-hsieh*; *chu-ling*—of each 3 mace. Dose: 8 mace, made into a decoction with water; no special time for taking it.

39. The True Jade Immortal's Method of Harmonizing the Hall of the Kidneys

To cure pain of the legs.

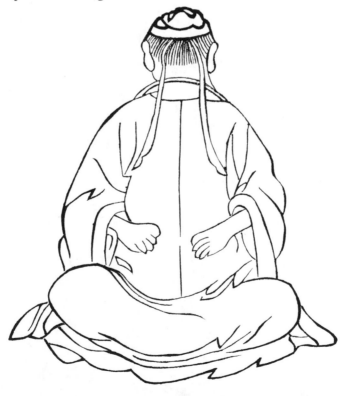

Sit upright; clench the two hands; rub them warm; place the palms of the hand to the posterior *ching* door; rub several times, the more the better, and each time revolve the air 24 times. (In spermatorrhea the legs are said to be painful.)

THE SOUP FOR REMOVING THE HEAT
AND OVERCOMING THE DAMP

Prescription Take of *huang-p'o* (moistened in salted water and afterwards roasted); *ch'iang-huo*; *tse-hsieh*; *ts'ang-shu*; prepared licorice (half the quantity of the other ingredients); *tu'chung* (roasted); *pai-shao* (roasted in wine); *mu-kua*; *wei-ling-hsien*; and orange peel—of each 1 mace; *niu-hsi* 牛 膝 —8 candareens. Add 3 slices of ginger, and make a decoction in water.

40. Li Yeh-p'o 李 埜 朴 Imitating the Child Reverencing
To cure the same as the preceding.

Sit firmly; extend both feet straight; use pressure to the root of the thighs; let the heart think and revolve the air 12 times.

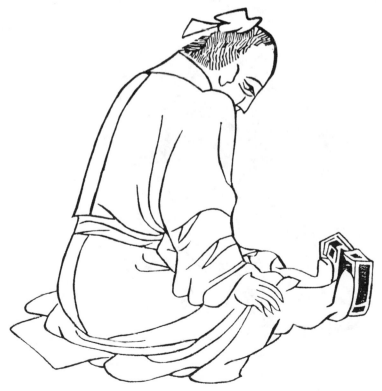

THE HAI-T'UNG-P'I POTION

Prescription Take *hai-t'ung-p'i*; *wu-chia-p'i*; *ch'uan-tu-huo*; *chih-ch'io*; *fang-feng*; *tu-chung* (roasted); *niu-hsi* (digested in wine); *i-i-jen* (roasted)—of each 1½ ounces. Put it into good wine, boil it to drive off the "fire" and the poison; to be taken on an empty stomach. Dose: 5 mace.

41. Lan Ts'ai-ho 藍 采 和 Imitating the Black Dragon Shaking His Horns

To cure pain of the entire body.

Lan Ts'ai-ho was one of the Eight Immortals, who wandered about a beggar in a tattered blue gown, with one foot shoeless, wearing wadded garments in summer and in winter sleeping on snow and ice. She waved a wand in her hand and chanted verses denunciatory of fleeting life and its delusive pleasures.

Sit upright; extend both feet; firmly close the two hands, and together with the body direct them to the front; revolve the air in 24 mouthfuls; place the feet on the ground; bend the head; let the two hands grasp the toes of the two feet; and revolve the air as above.

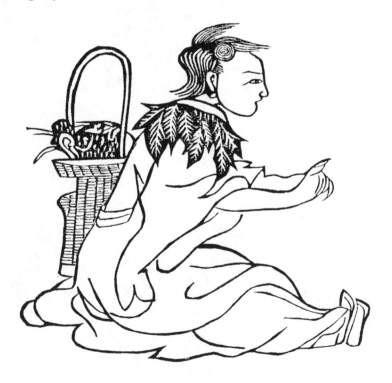

THE SOUP TO CAUSE THE BLOOD VESSELS TO CIRCULATE

Prescription Take of hsuan-hu-so; tang-kuei, and mou-kuei—of each 1 ounce. Powder and mix with wine. Dose: 3 or 4 mace. Add wine according to each individual's wine capacity; when the pain ceases, cease the medicine.

42. Hsia Yun-feng 夏 雲 峰 Imitating the Black Dragon in a Horizontal Position on the Ground

To cure pain of the back and spine.

Bend the body; creep on the ground; kneel; place the two hands on the ground; revolve the air right and left 6 times.

A similar exercise is enjoined in that known as Using the Golden Block to Sodden the Earth: for the cure of abdominal pain.

Both hands are raised above the head with the palms upwards as if supporting heaven, and both heels are pressed firmly on the ground; the arms are drawn down, and nine respirations are taken. [Compare number 7 of the Ornamental Sections]

THE TRINITY OR THREE HARMONIES SOUP

Prescription Take of orange peel; *pan-hsia*; *fu-ling*; *wu-yao*; *chih-ch'io*; *ch'uan-hsiung*; *pai-chih*; *ch'iang-huo*; *fang-feng*; *hsiang-fu*—of each the same quantity, and make a decoction.

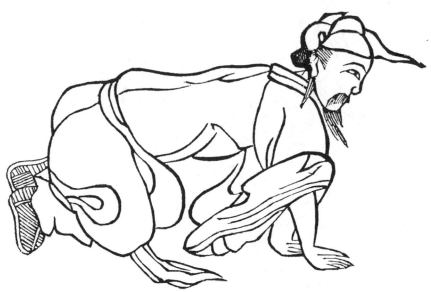

43. Ho T'ai-ku Supporting Heaven, Seated

To cure swelling of the abdomen from debility.

The above is sometimes called Supporting the Pagoda toward Heaven: for the cure of enlargement of the abdomen. (Compare this with standing Figure number 11 of Chang Tzu-yang Driving the Pestle.)

Seated upright, raise the two hands as if supporting something; move the air; and by upheaval lead the air upwards in 9 mouthfuls, then make it descend in 9 mouthfuls.

THE FRAGRANT SHA LING AND P'I POTION

Prescription Take of *fu-ling-p'i; ta-fu-p'i; wu-chia-p'i;* ginger-skin; *sang-pai-p'i; chih-ch'io; sha-jen; pai-shu; lo-fu-tzu; mu-hsiang; mu-t'ung; tse-hsieh; chu-ling*—of each the same quantity. Boil; to be taken a little while after meals.

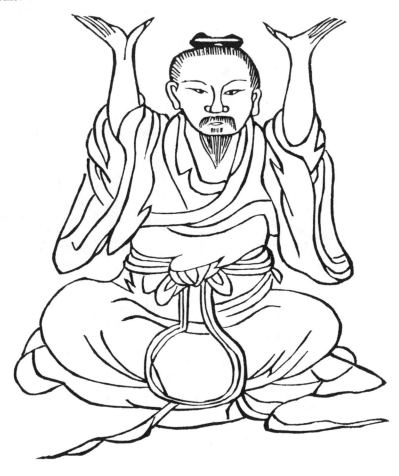

44. Liu Hsi-ku 劉 希 古 Exhibiting Terribly the Ferocious Tiger

To cure dysentery.

Place the two hands in front and behind (one in front, the other behind), like grasping a horse and putting aside flowers; place the feet also in front and behind, and take steps in performing the exercise. For white dysentery, let the air advance directed to the left in 9 mouthfuls; for red dysentery, the same to the right.

THE YELLOW WAX PILLS

Prescription Take of yellow wax—1 ounce; 49 almonds, digested in water to strip off the skin and the point [the latter supposed to be poisonous]; *mu-hsiang*—5 mace; and 7 croton seeds, Croton Tiglium (fold them in paper and beat to express the oil). Melt the wax, and mix in the ingredients to make pills the size of green peas. Dose: 15 for red dysentery, to be taken with licorice soup; for the white variety, use ginger as a menstruum.

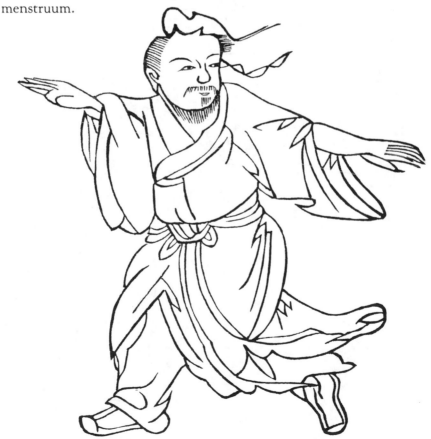

45. Miss Sun Pu-erh 孫 不 二 Waving the Flag

To cure the same as the preceding.

Direct the body to the front; extend the two hands straight in front as if taking hold of something; raise the right foot, so as to have the heel off the ground; then flex and extend the feet; revolve the air in 24 mouthfuls. Right and left the same.

THE PAI SHAO YAO SOUP

Prescription Take of *pai-shao*; and *tang-kuei*—of each 1 mace; rhubarb—2 mace; *mu-hsiang*—5 candareens; *huang-lien*—1mace; *huang-ch'in*; and betel-nut—of each 8 candareens; and licorice—7 candareens. For one dose. A decoction.

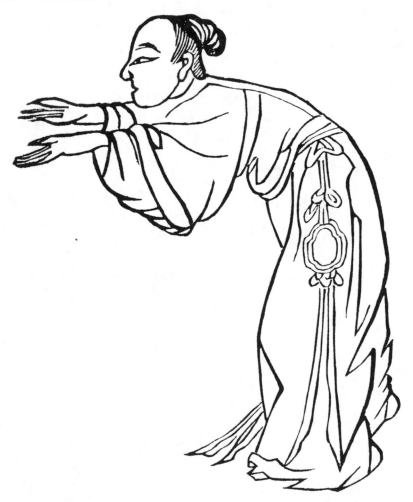

46. Ch'ang Yao-yang 常 天 陽 Imitating the Child Worshipping the Goddess of Mercy

To cure pain in front and back of heart.

The body is to assume the Chinese figure 8 (八); bend the head as far as the front of the chest; place the two hands on the abdomen; and revolve the air 19 times.

THE SOUP OF THE TWO ORANGES

Prescription Take of *chih-so* (same as *so-sha-mi*), Amomum villosum; *pan-hsia*; orange peel; *chih-shih*; *sha-jen*; *hsiang-fu*; *pai-hsiang*; *hou-p'o*; *hui-hsiang*; *hsuan-hu-so*; *ts'ao-tou-k'ou* 草 豆 蔻 ; *tzu-su* (stem and leaves)—of each the same quantity. Add 3 slices of ginger, and make a decoction.

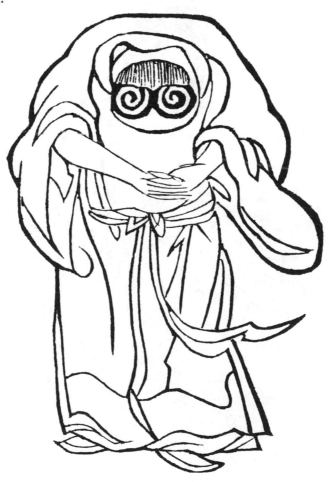

47. Tung-fang Shuo's 東 方 朔 Method of Grasping His Big Toes

To cure hernia.

It is related that Tung-fang Shuo (2nd century B.C.) was the child of a miraculous conception, and his mother removed to a place farther to the eastward from her home to give birth to her child; hence his name. According to common repute, he was the embodiment of the planet Venus. [Ed. note: He was also a famous Taoist-magician.]

With the two hands grasp the big toes of the two feet; bend the toes for a period equal to 5 respirations; lead the air in the abdomen throughout the entire body.

Another method is bending all the ten toes in this manner, which is better.

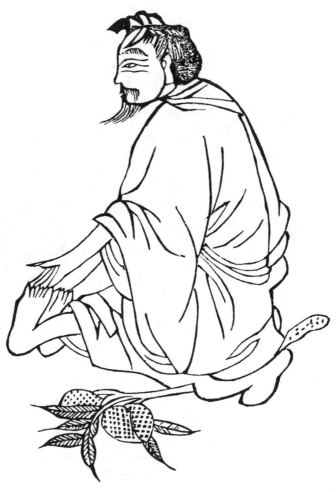

HUEI-HSIANG PILLS

Prescription Take *fu-ling; pai-chu; shan-ch'a*—of each 1 ounce; *chih-shih*—8 mace; *ta-huei-hsiang* (roasted)—1 ounce; *wu-chu-yu* 吳 茱 萸 (roasted)—1 ounce; orange seed (roasted)—2 ounces; *li'chih-ho* 荔 枝 核 , stones of Nephelium Litchi—1 ounce. Powder; form pills with honey, each pill to weight 1½ mace. To be taken on an empty heart [stomach]. Break up the pills and take with soup of ginger.

48. The Patriarch P'eng's 彭 祖 Method of Brightening the Vision

The Patriarch P'eng is a mythical being, who is reputed to have attained a fabulous longevity. He was 767 years of age when the Yin (Shang) dynasty came to an end (1123 B.C.). He is said to have nourished himself upon the powder of mother-o'-pearl and similar substances. He is regarded by some as one of the incarnations of Lao-tzu.

Sit on the ground firmly; reverse the two hands and place them behind; extend the left leg; flex the right knee and press it upon the left leg equal to a period of 5 respirations; and induce the lungs to drive out the wind. If this attitude be assumed for a long time, things at night will be seen as clear as day.

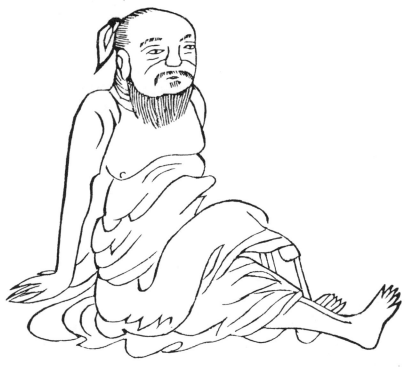

Another method is at cock-crow to rub the two hands warm, and iron (as it were) the eyes; rub thrice, and iron the eyes as often; then take the finger and rub the eyes, and right and left will become divinely brilliant.

THE TI-HUANG PILLS FOR CLEARING THE EYES

Prescription Take of *sheng-ti* (washed in wine); *shu-ti* (the same)—of each 4 ounces; *chih-mu* (roasted in salted water); *huang-po* (roasted in wine)—of each 2 ounces; cakes of *t'u-ssu-tzu* 兎 絲 子 , Cuscuda (Dodder) seeds (prepared in wine); *tu-huo*—of each 1 ounce; *kan-kou-chi*; *ch'uan-niu-hsi* (washed in wine)—of each 3 ounces; *sha-yuan-chi-li* 沙 苑蒺藜, seeds of an unknown plant—3 ounces. Powder, and make pills with honey the size of the *wu-t'ung-tzu* (seeds of Sterculia platanifolia). Dose: 80 pills. In summer, use weakly salted water as a menstruum. After more than a month, use wine in taking it.

These exercises conclude with a description of three Figures. The first Figure is a pipe or reed which is introduced into the two nostrils 3 *fen* deep. In calibre it must fit the nostrils exactly, so as to allow no leakage of air. The tube is pervious, and the apex has an aperture for blowing into. It is employed in constant coughing, in profuse perspiration, when the body is hot, the voice hoarse or lost, and in loss of flesh and constitutional weakness. In the case of haemoptysis, a cure is guaranteed in seven days by its use. It is only necessary to *hem* or flow into the tube.

To cure red sputum, each time the instrument is used, [prepare] a small cupful of *hsiang-ch'an* 香 蟾 [a venereal medicine, very costly and highly esteemed, said to be produced from a toad's forehead, and

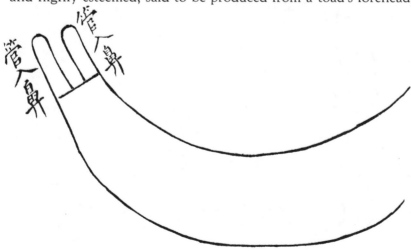

coming from the south]; mother's milk; two eggs; and a pig's pancreas cut very fine. Mix the whole thoroughly, then put it in a porcelain vessel or silver winecup. Steam it until well done, and take it every morning for seven days on an empty stomach at the same time as blowing into the pipe.

The second Figure is designed against fullness of the chest and weakness of the air (constitution). The instrument is to be placed on the navel. It will cure amenorrhea and spermatorrhea.

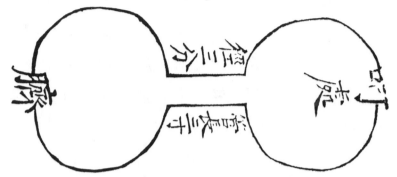

Before blowing into it, take 3 li of musk; gum olibanum—1 mace; catechu; myrrh; and sandalwood—of each 1 mace. Powder, and form into cakes with honey, one cake to be applied to the navel. Take 1 slice of ginger, the size of the cake and half the thickness of a cash [Chinese copper money]; take the artemisia (Tanacetum Chinense) and make into a pill or tuft the size of a bean [number unimportant], and burn until the ginger is hot. When the heat is felt inside, remove the medicine and blow into the instrument. No second application is necessary.

The third Figure is an instrument to be inserted two fen into the meatus urinarius, for the cure of spermatorrhea; it should be introduced smeared with wax. The blowing into it is to be according to the age of the patient, one blow for each year; the number may be increased, but not diminished.

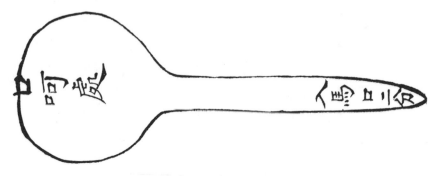

From 5 to 7 days before commencing the use of the instrument, whether the patients be male or female, the body is to be strengthened by the use of good wine, flesh and rice, that the improvement may be speedy.

[Ed. note: The author does not translate the rest of the instructions, but reproduces the original Chinese. The Chinese and a translation of the passage follow.]

若男子病，用童女。女人病，用童男。人壯盛無病者呵之。若丈夫病呵，用女人，女人病呵用男人亦可。

If it is a man who is ill, use a young girl; if a woman is ill, use a young boy. This person, who is healthy and without sickness, blows into it [the instrument]. If an older man is ill, use a woman to blow; if a woman is ill, using a man is also fine.

In the fourth Figure [illustration not included] (a tube resembling a rib), the patient reclines on the back with warm water or olibanum wine in the mouth; afterwards a young man is to blow into the tube according to the above directions. The following is the method.

Take red lead [a preparation made from menstrual discharge, and so called because of its resemblance to red lead], etc.

[Ed. note: Again, the author leaves the instructions in Chinese. The original passage and its translation follow.]

吹法先取紅鉛，用破身童女所行經脉，以夏布揉洗令淨，或淨花亦可。臨用時將熱童便洗下，晒乾，晒乾收起。用時以童便化開，滴於纂篇小頭口邊入鼻內，將大頭令童口便力吹之，如上法，病人候氣引入童女氣。

The method of blowing is to first procure "red lead" [see above]. Use blood which comes from a deflowered virgin; rub it into grass cloth and rinse it until pure . . . After binding it up, dry it in the sun until the time of use. After clarifying the heated urine of a youth, dry it in the sun and put it aside. Near the time of use, blend it together with the youth's urine.

A portion is dropped into the small end of the tube and placed in the nose; the youth then blows into the other end with all his force; the sick person waits until he experiences the *t'ung-nu-ch'i* (female fluid). Onions and garlic and all sorts of acid and acrid things are to be avoided. This plan, if followed for a long time, will add to one's longevity. If, after using the method, warmth is felt inside, mother's milk may be drunk.

功夫 Curative Kung Without Prescriptions

1. The Etiquette of the Immortals: for the cure of paralysis. Sit on a high seat, the left foot placed on the opposite thigh, and the right extended forwards; clasp both hands, and, with the head turned in one direction, stretch out the clasped hands in the other, and *vice versa*, inspiring 24 times.

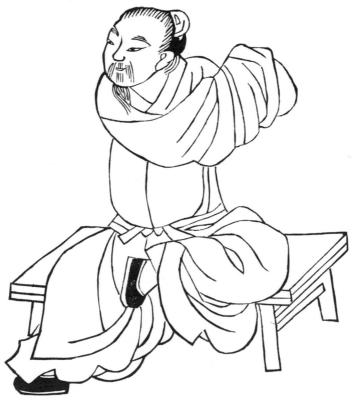

2. For the cure of lumbago and sciatica. Both hands together, bend them to the ground slowly; raise them up again quietly, straight above the head; shut the mouth, and breathe through the nose 3 or 4 times.

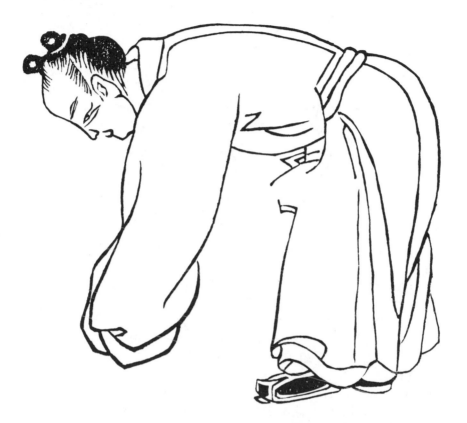

3. For the cure of cold of the kidneys, with pain in the back and limbs. Both hands are made warm and pressed against the lumbar region.

4. Li Po Enjoying the Moonlight: for the cure of stoppage of the blood. The position is like beating a serpent. Grasp the feet with the hands, reverse the hands, and take 12 breaths.

5. The Patriarch Lu's Method for Separating the Air: for the cure of stiffness of the body. With closed fists, press on both ribs on a level with the hollow of the breast [the ensiform cartilage at the bottom of the heart], and use strength internally in breathing 24 times on both sides.

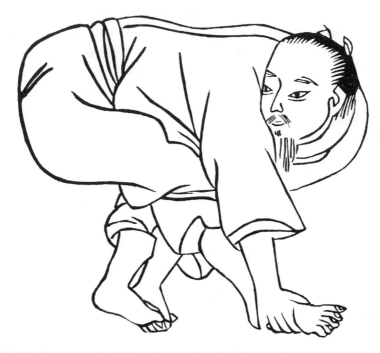

6. To harmonize the blood vessels, the three divisions of the body
   [upper, middle and lower parts of the trunk], and to cure indistinctness of vision and weakness. Sit cross-legged and rub the hands till
   warm, and then rub the soles of the feet; then press both hands on
   the knees, open the mouth, and inspire deeply 9 times.

7. Pa Wang's Walking Method: for the cure of painful contraction of
   the whole body caused by cold. Stand, and press closely with the
   hands upon the part above the crest of the ilium, first on one side,
   then on the other, in three positions, with one leg forward. Repeat
   12 times. (See Dragon Series, number 2)

功夫 Kneading

Under this title we include all forms of friction, pressing, rubbing, shampooing, massage, pinching, etc. This method for the cure and prevention of disease is of very ancient origin. It has been revived in modern times and is of growing importance, the practice being employed in a large and ever-increasing number of diseases. From times immemorial the department of pressing and rubbing, *An-mo-k'o* 按 摩 科 , has been one of the thirteen divisions of the great Medical College of China. This mode of treatment is used when the skin, tendons and muscles are injured or when the bones are fractured, or dislocated, or where the soft parts are swollen, hard or anaesthetic. If the vessels become pervious and the air is no longer blocked up, this method acts as a deiscutient and the disease is cured. The prevention and cure of disease by rubbing existed long anterior to the Founder of Taoism. Its place seems afterwards to have been taken by charms, incantations, magic and prayers, all of which, along with Kung-fu, alchemy and the elixir of immortality, are treated together in the Taoist books.

In the volume from which we have taken the "divine" Surgeon Hua-to's "Five Animals," there is the following on Shampooing (pressing and rubbing), called the Indian Method or That of Solomon, from the Sanskrit *sala* (*Shorea robusta*) the immense tree under which Buddha was born and died.

Grasp the hands and twist them as if washing them. Slightly interlock the hands and turn them backwards and forwards towards the breast. Grasp the hands and press them alternately on the right and left thigh.[1] Let the hands act on both sides as if drawing a bow of 5 piculs'

---

[1]The *pi* 髀 which occurs frequently in these directions for Shampooing is the thigh. It is the same as *pi* 脾 which is the same as *pi* 髀 , the thigh. *Pi ch'ih* 髀 胢 is the stomach.

resistance. With both hands press heavily on the thigh and slowly hoist the body on both sides. With firmly closed fists push the hands forward alternately. Stretch the fists upwards and downwards alternately to open the thorax. Act as if supporting a stone on the palm. Turn the hands backwards and strike the back on each side. Lay the hands on the ground and tilt up the body by bending the spine thrice. Embrace the head with the hands and turn it on the thigh. This is to pull out the shoulders. Sit sideways on the two sides alternately as if leaning against a hill. Sit and stretch out the feet alternately and draw them forward in space. Lay the hands on the ground and look backward on the right and left alternately. This is termed "tiger looking." Stand on the ground and twist the body round thrice. Deeply interlock the hands and tread the feet alternately in them. Stand erect and with the feet tread right and left in space. Sitting, stretch out the legs and hook them alternately at the knees.

These eighteen forms are to be practised thrice daily, and after one month even an aged person will become strong and run as fast as a horse, will be able to eat, will have bright eyes, and, moreover, will never feel tired or contract illness.

THE PRESSING AND RUBBING METHOD OF LAO-TZU

Press down heavily on the thigh with the hands on each side and twist the body twice seven (14) times. Press the thigh with the hands on each side and twist the shoulder twice seven (14) times. Embrace the head with the hands and twist the loins twice seven (14) times. Shake the head twice seven (14) times and support it thrice. Embrace the head with one hand and support the knee with the other and bend the body thrice on each side. Support the head with one hand and the knee with the other from below directed upwards, three times on each side. Grasp the head directed downwards with the hands and stamp the feet three times. Grasp the hands and pass them over the head right and left three times. Interlock the hands, support the heart in front [front of the breast], pushing out and turning them back three times. Interlock the hands and press the heart three times. Bend the wrist, buttress the ribs and draw back the elbow thrice on each side. Draw back the right and left side; pull forwards and backwards each three times. Extend the hands; draw back the neck thrice on each side. Lay the back of one hand on the knee and let the other draw back the elbow, then lay the palm on the knee three times on each side. Let the hand press the shoulder from above downwards and change the hands on each side. Push [the air] with the empty fists [loosely closed], three times. Interlock the hands and move them backwards and forwards reversing the dorsa and palms three times. Move the hands outwards, inwards and downwards each thrice. Rub and twist the finger thrice. Shake the hands backwards [reversing the dorsa and palms] three times. Interlock the hands and hoist the elbow up and down times without number and exhale the breath ten times only. Place the two hands together three times. Lower the two hands three times. Interlock the hands and pass them over the head; expand the ribs on the right and left ten times. Turn the fists backwards and rub the spine up and down three times. Turn the hands and grasp the ridge straight up and down three times.

Pronate the palm, take hold of the wrist and move it inwards and outwards thrice. Pronate the palm and interlock the two hands and move them horizontally three times. Pronate the palm in a straight horizontal position and lift them up three times. If the hands get cold, beat them from above downwards until they become warm. Extend the left foot and support it with the right hand, the right and left taking hold of the foot from above downwards, and straighten the foot three times. Let the right hand take hold of the foot, the same as the other. Whirl the foot backwards and forwards three times. Whirl the foot to the left and to the right, each three times. Whirl the foot backwards and forwards three times. Straighten the feet three times. Twist the thigh three times. Shake the foot inwards and outwards three times. If the foot gets cold, beat it until warm. Twist the thigh so many times and stamp the feet three times and straighten them three times. Act like a tiger on the right and left and twist the shoulder three times. Push the heavens and support the earth right and left three times. Swing a mountain [like a pendulum] right and left, carry a hill [on the back], and pull up a tree, each three times. Extend the hands and twist them straight in front three times, knees and feet each three times. Twist the spine inwards and outwards, each thrice. [For further remarks on this method see further on.]

The patriarch Peng says that by rubbing the face and ears with the hands every morning, the vigour of the face will then flow everywhere. Again, by rubbing the hands until they get warm, and then rubbing the face, the latter will look bright and be able to bear the cold without suffering.

He also says that the person who wishes to harmonize the breath must take a room, shutting the window and door, with a warm mat and a high pillow. With the body reclining perfectly straight, shut up the eyes and the breath in the chest, and put a feather on the nose so that it does not move. After 300 breaths, the eyes will not see, the ears will not hear [will become insensible], neither cold nor heat will come nigh the body, and no poisonous insects will deposit their virus on it; the person will attain to the age of 360 years and thus become a neighbor of the Immortals.

Every morning and evening with the face towards the South, place the hands on the feet and the knees, knead the joints gently, exhale the foul breath by the mouth, and inhale the pure air by the nose; with the hands right and left, support the abdomen in front and behind, above and below. After awhile, open the mouth, knock the teeth, wink the eyes, press the head, pull the ears, curl up the hair, loose the loins and cough in order to develop and excite the breath. Turn the hands, and using the idea stamp the feet eighty or ninety times and then stop. Settle the heart slowly, preserve the thought like a Buddhist priest, shut the eyes and you will then see the original air come gradudally down as a canopy of (3) distinctly different colours to the head, pass through the skin to the flesh, the bones, the brain and finally to the abdomen; all the inferior viscera will derive benefit from it like the absorption of water. When the *ku-ku* noise is heard in the abdomen, then keep the thought and do not let it communicate with external things, so the original air will be transported to the "sea of air" 氣 海, and finally to the *yung ch'uan* 勇 泉 [acupuncture aperture on the inner aspect of the sole of the foot between the heel and great toe], and the body will be excited.

It is to be done once or twice a day up to as many as three to five times; the effect will be that the body will feel pleasant, the face appear bright and the hair glossy, the ear and the eye will become clear and intelligent, and the strength of the air will become robust and all diseases will be removed. If it could be performed 5,000 or 10,000 times without stopping, up to the full 100,000 times, the Kung-fuist is not far from the Immortals.

And thus it comes about that the body is full of the suitable air free from sickness; otherwise all manner of disease will be engendered. Whoever, therefore, wants to improve his health must know how to harmonize the breath. It may be held after midnight and before noon, when the air is alive and can be profitably harmonized; in the afternoon or before midnight the air is dead and unprofitable. Lie on the back on thick, warm bedding and a high pillow, keep the body even, stretch out the hands and feet, bend the joints of the thumb 4 or 5 inches apart from the body and the feet the same distance apart from each other, knock the teeth frequently and swallow the saliva, breathe air through the nose into the abdomen until full; after awhile, gradually exhale from the mouth and repeat the process continuously. Where there is a heavy fog, or bad wind and extreme cold, the breath should not be inhaled. When one has caught a cold and is feverish or has malignant boils, the *kung* must be performed at once, no matter what the time may be, and continued until one is cured.[2]

Another of the Taoist patriarchs, Ju Hsu, says that at cock crowing we should rise, sit on the bed and guide [refine] the breath; when finished and our toilet is completed, we should sit straight and, according to whether the season is cold or hot, take some refreshment. Before we partake, a little medicinal wine is to be drunk. After it has dispersed, enter some quiet place, burn incense and purify the heart, after which read or chant prayers or charms and thoroughly wash away every thought of anger, grief, care, etc., from the heart. After a little while, go out into the courtyard and slowly take step after step, letting off the breath. If the ground is damp the walking must be intermitted. Take five steps outside the room to disperse the air. Pass the management of all domestic affairs to your son, and thus set the heart free from all family cares. If the heart cannot be made and kept pure at home, then seek a retreat elsewhere, whether 50 or 100 *li* distant, and daily contemplate peace; whatever is needed there, let some of the family bring it, etc.

The patriarch Shih-shih says: After meals first rub the abdomen with a warm hand and walk fifty or sixty steps; repeat the operation after the midday meal and walk one hundred or two hundred steps, but never walk hastily to cause panting. Return to the couch and lie down, extend the limbs but do not sleep; after the breath becomes settled, sit up and take some medicinal articles such as dates, ginseng, China-root and licorice in a decoction. When a degree of warmth is experienced, take a decoction of bamboo leaves, *imperata arundinacea* (*ophiopogon japonicus*). When the stomach is full do not walk quickly, and when it is empty do not use the voice to call or use one's breath.

The patriarch Chung Cheng says that man ought not only to know how to take his proper food but also how to harmonize the body by rubbing and kneading, moving the joints and guiding the breath. The importance of the latter is to keep the breath moving so as not to become an obstruction.

I intended to describe the shampooing, rubbing, pressing, and other

[2]Extreme caution is advised, and this should only be practiced by the initiated.

processes of the fraternity of barbers for the cure of disease, the prolongation of life in the healthy, the production of a sense of comfort and the removal of fatigue, etc., but considerations of space render it necessary to pass over this part of Kung-fu. A small illustrated book in two volumes, The Barber's Classic, entitled Ching-fa-hsü-chih 淨 髮 須 知, or "how to obtain clean hair," may be profitably consulted. The second volume treats, in part, massage applied to the various parts of the body. It also treats the acupuncture apertures, a knowledge of which is essential to the proper practice of the art. It speaks of 84,000 pores, of 10 ching and 15 lo (arterial vessels), and of the merit accruing from the exercise of this method, which is modified by certain climatic and physical conditions, such as the state of the weather, whether cold or hot, and the condition of the patient, whether fat or lean, etc. The sections embrace massage in general, and rubbing as applied to the apertures of the back and loins, hands and arms, head and face, thorax and abdomen, and lower limbs.

On the streets of the Capital there is a class of masseurs whose art is known as tien-p'i 點 皮 ("pressing the skin"). The generic name of the class is t'ui-na 推 拿 . For example, for the cure of pain in the temples, the part below the sternum is pressed; for the cure of cold and pain, the part below the ribs; for colic, the points of the fingers and lips; for headache, the shoulders; for toothache, the facial artery, shoulder, the cleft of thumb and forefinger; for cholera, the calf of the leg; for general discomfort, the blood vessels.

功夫 Divisions of The External Method

Each of the following *kung-fu* exercises focuses energy on a separate part of the body.

HEART

While performing the exercise one must first rest the mind, cease from all thought, banish all grief, anger and suchlike, and give up all the animal propensities, in order to keep and not disperse the vital essence.[1]

BODY

When sitting crosslegged, the heel of one foot must block up the perineum and not allow the vital spirits to leak out.

Sit evenly; the knees must be level with the body, and the "sons of the kidney" must not rest on the seat but hang down. (*Note:* Sitting high and level refers to sitting on chairs and beds.)

After finishing the exercise and rising, the limbs must be slowly extended, and on no account should this be done hastily.

In sitting, the body must be level and straight, the spinal column must be perpendicular and not bent, and one must not lean against anything on the right or left.

HEAD

Close the ears with the hands, let the second (fore) finger fold itself on

[1]One author recommends, with the view of prolonging life, employing oneself in such thoughts and designs as lead to virtue—to reflect often on the happiness of our lot, to seek to know the value of health, and to study to preserve it. Once in bed, lull the heart (mind) to sleep by composing it, throwing aside thoughts that would banish sleep. The heart will be kept in good condition and the dissipation of the vital and animal spirits prevented if, while in bed, we lie on either side with the knees bent a little.

the middle one, and thrum the two bones at the back of the skull with the second finger to make them sound. This is called sounding the "heavenly drum." (*Note:* This is to remove the vicious air from the "wind pool" acupuncture opening in the region of the mastoid.)

Twist the neck with the hands and glance back to the right and left, and at the same time rotate the shoulders and arms, each 24 times. To remove the obstructed air in the stomach and spleen.

Interlock the hands and grasp the back of the neck, then look upwards and let the hands wrestle with the neck. To remove pain of the shoulders and indistinctness of vision.

FACE

Rub the hands until hot, then rub the face with them, high and low, all over, no spot to be left unrubbed; then spit on the palms, rub them warm, and apply them several times to the face. While rubbing, the breath is to be closed by the mouth and nose. The aim of this exercise is to brighten the countenance—the more you rub the better the colour. This is the cure for wrinkles; with this action you will have none.

EAR

Place the hands over the ears, then rub them right and left and up and down several times. This is to hear distinctly and prevent deafness.

Sit level on the ground with one leg bent and the other extended. Stretch forth the arms horizontally with the hands perpendicular towards the front, as if pushing a door; twist the head seven times to each side. To cure ringing in the ears.

EYE

When you awake, do not open the eyes, but rub the back of the thumbs until they become hot, then wipe the eyes with them fourteen times; still keeping the eyes shut, rotate the eyeballs to each side seven times. Shut them tightly for a little while and then suddenly open them wide. This is to protect the "divine light" and to remove disease from the eye forever. Rubbing the thumbs hot on the palm of the hand will also do.

Use the bent bone of the thumb [ungual phalanx] and press heavily on the little apertures at the sides of the eyebrows [temples] $3 \times 9 = 27$ times. Again rub the malar bones and round the pinna of the ear 30 times with the two hands. Again let the hands press upon the frontal region 27 times, beginning between the two eyebrows and proceeding backwards to the margin of the hair at the back of the head; swallow the saliva times without number. To give clearness and brightness to the eyes and ears.

Place the hands on the inner canthi of the eyes near the root of the nose; shut up the breath, and when the air has become pervious, stop. By doing this constantly, objects will be seen very distinctly, obstructions in the nose will be removed, and coryza may also be cured in this way.

When kneeling or sitting, let the hands touch the ground and turn the head in order to take a backward glance 5 times. This is termed the "Tiger's glance." To remove the vicious wind of the thorax and kidneys. This exercise can be carried out in bed; the hands need not necessarily be placed on the ground.

MOUTH

When performing the exercise, the mouth must be closed.

When there is great dryness and bitterness of the mouth, the tongue is rough, and one is swallowing without saliva; when one has pain in the pharynx, whether in swallowing or expectorating and inability to eat, this is owing to inflammation [heat]. The mouth must be opened wide, the air blown [hemmed] over a dozen times, the "heavenly drum" sounded 9 times, and the tongue must excite the saliva; blow again and then swallow. Wait till the "pure water" [saliva] is produced, and the heat will be driven back and the viscera cooled. Again, if the saliva in the mouth is cold and without taste, and the heart feels as if it contained water, this is owing to cold; one must take the air and warm it. Wait until the mouth has recovered its taste; the cold is disarmed and the viscera warmed.

Every morning gently breathe out the foul air from the mouth, and at the same time take in the pure air by the nose and swallow it.

In sleeping, shut the mouth; do not let the original constitutional air come out and corrupt air enter.

TONGUE

Place the tongue against the roof of the mouth in order to excite the saliva and fill the mouth, then rinse the mouth 36 times and swallow it in three mouthfuls, making the gurgling sound ku-ku in the pharynx. The saliva entering the abdomen will moisten the viscera.

TEETH

Knock the teeth 30 times to collect the spirits.

During micturition shut the mouth and press the teeth firmly. To remove toothache.

NOSE

Rub the thumbs of the two hands until they become hot, then rub the nose with them 36 times. To moisten the lungs.

Let the eyes look at the point of the nose and then breathe silently several times.

Every evening, lie prone in bed with the pillow removed, bend the legs while keeping the feet upright, inhale the pure air by the nostrils 4 times, and expire by the nose 4 times. In expiration use energy; afterwards breathe gently by the nose. To cure heat of the body and pain of the back.

HAND

Interlock the hands, support the empty void of heaven with the palms, and lay them on the head 24 times, to remove the vicious air of the thorax.

Let one hand be stretched forward and the other bent backward as if drawing a very tight bow, equal to a resistance of 500 catties. To remove the vicious air of the arms and asillae.

Tightly clench the two hands and strike the arms and thighs with the fists; then turn the hands backwards and strike the back—each 36 times. To remove the vicious air of the four pits [the two axillae and the two groins].

Hold the fists tightly, bend the elbows backwards, draw them backwards 7 times, and let the head twist and follow the hands to the right and left. To cure red boils of the body.

Let the two fists strike the emptiness with energy right and left 7 times. To remove [strike the emptiness with energy] the vicious wind of the thorax.

FEET

Sitting upright, stretch the feet, bend the head as if worshipping, and with energy let the hands grasp the soles 12 times. To remove the vicious air of the pericardium.

Sitting on a high place with the feet hanging down, let the heels be rotated opposite each other outwards, and let the toes converge opposite each other inwards, each 24 times. To cure rheumatism of the feet.

Seated crosslegged, take hold of the toes with one hand and rub the sole with the other until it becomes hot. In the sole there is the "bubbling fountain" aperture from which damp and wind find exit; when the sole is rubbed hot, this may stop, then move the toes themselves. To cure dampness and heat and increase the walking energy.

Kneeling on one leg, the hands supported by the bed, extend and flex the legs alternately 7 times. Change from right to left. To remove swelling of the knees and ankles.

Clench the fists slowly, step with the left foot to the front, pronate and supinate the left hand in front and the right behind; in the same manner do it on the right. To remove the vicious air of the two shoulders.

SHOULDER

Set the shoulders in a rotatory motion with the hands, turning the windlass alternately right and left, 24 times. First rotate the left, then the right; this is termed the "Single Pulley." Then rotate both together; this is called the "Double Pulley."

Rest and harmonize the mind, rub the navel with each hand alternately 14 times, then the ribs and shoulders 7 times, inspire, and convey the air to the *tan-t'ien*; clench the fists tightly and lie down on one side, bending the feet. To prevent nocturnal emissions.

BACK

Let the hands rest on the bed, contract (shrink) the body in a heap, bend the back, bow the vertebra column, and raise it up 13 times. To remove the vicious air of the heart and liver.

ABDOMEN

Rub the abdomen with the hands and walk one hundred steps. To cure indigestion.

Close the breath and think the fire of the *tan-t'ien* up to burn the whole body.

LOINS

Hold the fists tightly, place them on the ribs, and shake the shoulders 24 times. To remove pain and vicious air from the loins.

Rub the hands hot, take a breath of pure air by the nose and gradually let it out, then with the warm hands rub the semen door, *i.e.*, the soft part below [at the lower part of] the back.

KIDNEYS

Grasp with one hand the "two sons" of the inside and outside kidneys [the Chinese suppose them connected], and with the other hand rub the navel, each hand 81 times. This instruction is put into a rhyme thus: one rub, one suspend, right and left change hands, nine times nine in number and the male principle will not go.

Before sleeping, sit on the bed with the legs hanging down, open the clothes, close the breath, apply the tongue to the roof of the mouth, and direct the eyes to the "door of the vertex" [the crown of the head]. Elevate and contract the "cereal road" as if to prevent defecation, and with the two hands rub the two apertures called *Shen-yü* of the two kidneys, each 120 times. To produce semen, strengthen the membrum virile, remove pain from the loins and prevent frequent micturition.

NOTES ON KUNG-FU REGULATING THE VARIOUS PARTS OF THE BODY

It will be observed that the cause of disease is invariably supposed to depend upon the presence of vitiated or depraved air, which has stealthily gained admittance. The air thus shut up causes obstruction. It is sometimes termed thievish air or air deflected from its proper course. The Chinese proverb runs: Avoid a draught of air as you would the point of an arrow. It is recommended that one rub the soles of the feet until hot and also move each toe, this measure being effectual in preserving and repairing the vital and animal spirits. The middle of the sole is supposed to be the outlet of a great many services of spirits, and, like mouths of rivers, the arteries and veins end there, and therefore must be kept open.

It is advisable, every time one awakes, to stretch oneself in bed, thus facilitating the course of the spirits and circulation. One ought not to sleep like a dead man (*i.e.*, not to lie on one's back), not to let the hands rest on the breast or heart, so as to avoid dreams and nightmares.

Once in bed one should keep silence and refrain from talking. The lungs are the most tender of the viscera and are consequently placed uppermost; they serve for respiration and promotion of the voice. When one takes any position in bed, they incline to rest upon that side; talking forces the lungs to partially raise themselves, and by strongly heaving, to shake the other noble internals parts. The voice comes from the lung as the sound from a bell; if the bell is not hung, it is damaged when struck to make it sound. Confucius never spoke after he was in bed; doubtless he made it a rule for this reason.

The Chinese have, as a rule, good teeth. The better classes use warm tea or water with which to cleanse them each morning and after meals. It is ordered to sleep with the head and face uncovered and with the mouth shut, as this tends to keep the radical moisture from escaping and preserves the teeth. Early loss of teeth is caused by the air passing in and out between them; besides, gross particles are inhaled, which give rise to distempers.

The *tan-t'ien* is situated about 1½ inches below the navel and is brought into exercise with the bow and arrow exercise. A person is said to be strong when this is in sufficient quantity.

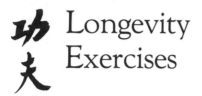 Longevity
Exercises

The following exercises remove disease and lengthen life.
1. Place the three middle fingers of the two hands in the "hollow of the heart" [depression below the ensiform cartilage, the heart of good people supposedly in the centre]. Beginning on the left side, rub round 21 times.

2. Same as number 1, but rub downwards to the high bone below the navel [pubic bone].

3. Same as number 2, but at the pubic bone divide the hands, rub up to the "heart hollow," bring the hands together again.

4. Same as number 3, but rub straight down at once to the pubic bone 21 times.

5. Rub with the right hand from the left round the navel 21 times.

6. Same as number 5, but rub with the left hand from the right side 21 times.

7. Place the left hand on the left loin, the thumb to the front, the four remaining fingers behind gently nipping the part; place the three middle fingers of the right hand below the left nipple and push down at once to the groin 21 times.

8. Same as number 7, but on the right.

9. The rubbing finished, sit crosslegged and let the thumbs of the hands press the *Tse* furrows [*i.e*, the base wrinkles of the 4th finger].[1]

[1]The Chinese reckon the 12 Earthly Branches beginning at this point, then going to the corresponding wrinkles of the middle and index fingers, then to the remaining two wrinkles on the forefinger with the apex, then to the apices of the next three fingers and the three remaining wrinkles of the little finger.

Then flex the four fingers, keeping the fingers apart; press the two knees; bend the toes; twist the thorax from the left to the front and from the right to the back, making in all 21 revolutions. When this is finished, perform from the right side, in a similar manner, 21 times. If you wish the body directed to the left according to the foregoing method, rotate the chest and shoulders outside the level of the left knee and rest them upon the left knee, and the right in like manner; then bend the back like a bow. Do not twist the loins too much, or too quickly, or with too much force. [The simple illustrations are omitted for want of space.]

In rubbing the abdomen, collect the spirits, empty the heart of all worldly affairs, let the pillow not be too high; the mat must be level. Lie flat on the back, the feet extended the same length; flex the fingers, and gently rub the abdomen. Go through the eight figures one after the other. This constitutes one course, which is to be performed 7 times; then rise, sit, and make 21 revolutions. Do this in the morning, at noon and in the evening; the first and last must not be neglected on any account. At the first *kung* take two courses; after three days, each *kung* must consist of 5 courses, and after another similar period each *kung* must comprise 7 courses. This is the rule for both sexes. In the parturient [pregnant] condition, the female is to intermit the exercises.

A work entitled *Fu-ch'i-ch'u-ping-t'u-shuo* 服 氣 祛 病 圖 說 (A Treatise, with plates, on Swallowing Air in the Cure of Disease) was published in 1846 and contains sixty-four illustrations. As active gymnastic exercises, not passive and contemplative, they might be introduced into our schools with profit. We give below the brief descriptions of the figures and regret that our space prevents the insertion of the diagrams.

The following eleven rules are laid down for the regulation of this art.

1. To swallow or gulp breath is of the first importance in the due performance of Kung-fu. Gulping breath [air] is different from disciplining or refining it; for if the latter is not well-performed, phlegm may obstruct and the "fire" may not descend. But this is the easier and is free from any disadvantage. In gulping, one must stand erect, look level, open the mouth wide and, as the true [original] air exists naturally in the body, so must the air be swallowed gently, as if drinking tea. At first there is no sound in swallowing; later a certain sound is produced which goes straight to the *tan-t'ien*, leading the "fire" to the original place. When the mouth is opened wide, it

should not be too small; otherwise the constitution will be injured by the wind which is inhaled.

2. Avoid hasty wind, violent rain, thunder and lightning; these are the anger of heaven and earth. Also dread impure and deflected air. Select a high, bright and clean room, not opposite to the wind.

3. Thrice daily—dawn (5–7 A.M.), noon (11 A.M.–1 P.M.), and twilight (5–7 P.M.)—perform these exercises without intermission. If business should interfere, then alter the time to either before or after the fixed period, say on rising and retiring independent of the hours, and for the midday exercises suit your own convenience. The *kung* must be performed on an empty stomach so that the air may freely circulate; if the stomach is full, the breath gets obstructed and injury may result. The sixty diagrams can be easily performed in half an hour. This is not a difficult task.

4. In swallowing air, the head is not to be directed upwards lest the bodily heat should rush upwards; neither should it be directed downwards, lest the breath sink. If these exercises are performed when one is fatigued, one will at once feel pleasant.

5. No matter whether one is ill or not, it is not necessary to take medicine, in case it should obstruct the breath. Even chronic bronchitis, dropsy, and inability to swallow food get well by the performance of these exercises. Three exercises daily must be gone through; neither more nor less will be found suitable. In exercising, the strength must not be over-exerted; it must be done, as it were, of itself.

6. At the commencement of these exercises, all drink and venery are to be avoided. Three months later this rule may be neglected. Weak persons should abstain from both of these throughout their entire lives.

7. These exercises may be performed by anyone, including women and children. If women practise them, they will have no difficult labours; their strength will be equal to that of men. The aged will become as strong as young people.

8. At the commencement, perform the "level frame position" by gulping the breath seven times; ten days after, add the first "military position," once on each side. Keep on practising in this manner for a month—*i.e.*, three times each ten days—thus performing the military position three times and gulping the air eighteen times. Ten days after these, perform the position of "resting on the knee" thrice

on each side and together gulp six mouthfuls of air. Then change the level position into the "moon-looking" one, a form of scooping up the moon [when reflected in water], omitting the two "expanding-breath" forms. Twenty days after this [in two periods of ten], the exercise termed the *chin-hsiao* (the standing digesting) form is to be performed twice on each side with twelve gulps of breath. The exercises have now been performed for eighty days, and forty-nine breaths have been swallowed. Hereafter the "beating" exercises are to be performed.

9. In beating, make a bag with a double blue cloth, 18 or 19 inches in length and 3 or 4 inches in circumference, like a girdle, one end closed and the other open. Pack it firmly with grain, 8 or 9 inches deep, tie the open end tightly with a piece of rope, and use the remaining half of the bag as a handle. The grain should weigh 2 catties. If the person is weak, diminish the amount.

10. In beating, first beat the left, then the right side of the body, and lastly the four surfaces of the hands and feet. Beat first from the inside of the left elbow down to the palm and then to the end of the middle finger. Then beat the outside in the same direction. Then beat from the left armpit down to the side of the fifth finger, and from the left shoulder down to the side of the thumb.

   After finishing beating the left upper limb, transfer the process to the left lower limb. First beat from the left ribs passing down the left side of the abdomen, then to the front of the leg to the knee, instep, dorsum of foot and left big toe. Then from the left axilla beat inclined to the left loin, passing to the outer ankle and turning to the side of the small toe. Then from the end of the breast bone (sternum) to the left side of the abdomen, and from the part which lies between the ribs and abdomen, pass horizontally to the right of the abdomen. Here change to the left hand in holding the bag, and from the right side beat horizontally to the left of the body. Let the right hand cover and protect the secret parts and let the left hand begin beating from the "little abdomen" and the inside of the left leg, passing down to the ankle and side of the toe.

   Then hold the bag with the two hands and raise it up over the head, beating the left part of the back twenty times; then hold the bag in the left hand and turn the hand and beat the underpart of the back, passing gradually down to the end of the lumbar region; then turn the hand and beat the left leg, down to the calf and heel.

After finishing the exercises on the left limbs, the right limbs are taken in hand in a similar manner.

The beating must be done closely from the upper to the lower part. No part is to be neglected nor any retrograde movement made. If a certain portion is neglected, it must not be repaired; the exercise must be steadily and continuously prosecuted. On beginning the beating, one breath is first taken, which makes altogether 16 mouthfuls of air, which, with the preceding 49, now reckons 65 in all.

After one or two months of beating, add the seven positions of the "inspecting-hand" and take four mouthfuls of breath. After ten days more add the "side-lifting" position, and take six mouthfuls of breath, then add the "front-lifting" position and take three more mouthfuls. After ten days more, perform the "Hsueh-kung standing" position and take three mouthfuls, and after another ten days exercise the "arranging-elbow" position and take six mouthfuls. Altogether we have now swallowed twenty-two mouthfuls of air, and this added to the previous 65 makes a total of 87 mouthfuls. These are the first part of the exercises.

11. Sixty-four diagrams are here described; they are only the first portion of the primary part of Kung-fu. If we count all of them, they exceed more than a thousand. In performing the first part, all diseases will disappear and one's vitality will be augmented two-fold. There remain still the second, third, and fourth parts, which will take two years to perform.

Since completing the *kung*, the pulse has gathered to the head; the body will possess the strength of 1,000 catties, sufficient, as is recorded in the *I-chin-ching*, to enable the fingers to pass simultaneously through the belly of an ox or to cut off the head of an ox with the edge of the palm. The advantage accruing is even greater than this. If these sixty-four positions are continually performed, the Kung-fuist will avoid disease and prolong his life. Speaking generally, diseases reside in the inner viscera and may be cured with medicine, but those which exist in the muscles and blood vessels cannot be reached by the power of drugs. If one wishes to secure ease to the muscles and blood vessels and prevent the air and blood from offering obstruction, except by the exercise of these *kung* no effect will be produced. Many people have experienced the beneficial results derived from the performance of these exercises.

This method was obtained from the province of Kuei-chou; it was delivered orally, and because this method is closely related to the *T'ai-*

hsi-tao-yin 胎息導引 [one of the Taoist doctrines and practices referred to in several sections in the work *Sheng-ming-kuei-chih*], the person does not desire to transmit it [in print], nor to have his name become known. Notwithstanding this, the method is profitable for physical improvement, and figures have been drawn and explanations made according to the oral explanations, and the work is now published. Let everyone therefore accept the advantage.

功夫 Description of Diagrams

THE LEVEL FRAME 平和架

There are four "horse-riding" 騎馬式 forms under this position.

1. Standing evenly and uprightly, separate the feet the width of the shoulders apart, and keep the palms upward on the same level as the loins. Do not lean against anything.

2. Turn the palms downwards, always on the same level as the loins.

3. Rub evenly from the sides and make a circle as if rubbing the head.

4. Then stretch the arms straight forward and erect the hands with the palms directed forward and fingers upwards on the same level as the nipple; take one breath and wait a little, about the time of three respirations. Then, after you have taken a breath, the eyes should be directed to the right, left, above, and below, the time of three respirations being taken as the unit.

There are also two "moon-looking" 望月式 forms under this position.

1. Let the left foot take a step horizontally to the side, bend the left knee, and incline the left foot; keep both the right leg and foot straight. Lay the left hand on the upper aspect of the thigh, with the thumb directed backwards, and wind the right hand round the back of the right ear with the five fingers in a form as if holding something, the points of the fingers directed backwards like the claws of a vulture.

2. Afterwards, raise the left hand up to the level of the eye, the fingers clenched so that the thumb is opposite the little finger, and the second, the fourth, and the middle one projecting a little. Keep the

palm—the heart of the hand—hollow, sufficient to contain the lid of a tea cup. First look at the height of the left hand, then turn the head even and take a breath. Again turn the head and look at the part between the thumb and forefinger. Repeat this on the right side—three times on each side, swallowing six mouthfuls of air.

There are two "expanding-breath" 舒 氣 式 forms under this position.

1. The first resembles the first "horse-riding" form, except that the palms are even.

2. The second resembles the last "horse-riding" form, except that the hands are turned and pushed to the front like the last of the "horse-riding" forms, and no breath is taken.

PRELIMINARY MILITARY EXERCISES 武 功 頭

There are three forms under this position, and seven diagrams.

1. The left foot bent, the right foot straight, the remainder the same as the first "moon-looking" position, and in addition with the face straight, take a breath and turn the head to the left.

2. Stretch out the left hand, which was formerly laid on the leg, straight to the left, keeping the palm downwards.

3. Turn the left hand back to the level of the breast, and then stretch it out again and bring it back, repeating two times.

4. Turn the hand over on the breast, with the thumb upwards, the other fingers downwards, and the palm opposite the breast, and take a breath.

5. Turn the hand with the thumb downwards and the middle finger upwards, and turn the head to the left.

6. Stretch out the hand opposite to the breast and wind it round the ear; keep the palm directed upwards and extend it to the left.

7. Turn it back from behind the ear and clench the fist in front of the breast; keep the outer part of the fist directed upwards, take a breath and then turn the head to the left. To be done on the right also—each side three times, altogether taking eighteen breaths.

THE CIRCULATING OR INSPECTING-HAND POSITION 巡 手

Standing erect, keep the feet 15 or 16 inches apart; extend the elbows forward evenly, the wrists straight and perpendicular to each other, and the fingers separated.

THE JADE GIRDLE POSITION 玉 帶

Separate the palms, pressing them down behind the ears to the loins on the level of the navel; keep the tips of the fingers apart and corresponding to each other, and distant from the body three inches, interlocking, as it were, the loins; take a breath.

THE SUSPENDING-LOIN POSITION 垂 腰

Apply the fists to the loins, turn the backs of the hands downward, and full in front take a breath.

THE HOLDING-UP ROBE POSITION 提 袍

Open the fists, turn them from the underpart of the ribs, pronate the palms and stretch them forward evenly as if lifting something, and full in front take a breath.

THE TURBAN POSITION 幞 頭

Separate the hands and turn them out from under the ribs to above the head to a distance of 7 or 8 inches from the head; direct the palms outwards, the fingers separated and opposite each other, with the thumb downwards on a level with the eyes.

THE BRUSHING-FACE POSITION 搔 面

There are two forms under this position.

1. Keep the palms of the hands close together in front of a level with the chin, and the two little fingers and elbows applied close together; raise them together over the forehead.

2. Gradually bend the fingers in order to make hooks of them, and then slowly clench the fists and place them under the chin; open them [the fists] again, bring the thumbs together, and extend the hands and pass them over the forehead; also keep the two little fingers together, and finally make the hands into fists and place them again under the chin. The wrists and elbows should be close together.

THE COURT TABLET POSITION 朝 笏

Pull the fists apart on a level with the shoulders, in a circular form as if enfolding things, the back of the hand directed upwards and the fists opposite each other, and apart 18 or 19 inches; and in front take a breath.

THE SIDE-LIFTING POSITION 偏 提

There are three forms under this position.

1. Standing aslant, the left foot bent, the right foot erect, interlock the hands and raise them with energy over the head.

2. Bend the body gradually as if making a bow, as far as the instep of the foot; turn the palms and press downwards; afterwards interlock them again and raise them to the space between the knee and the chin; then all at once make a whirl, and straighten the body and loins.

3. Separate the hands and let them circle round the ears, then clench the fists and bend the arms in a circular form; the two fists opposite each other and 18 or 19 inches apart, and the back of the hands kept upwards, take a breath. It is done in the same way on the right —thrice on each side, taking altogether six breaths.

THE FRONT-LIFTING POSITION 正 提

There are three forms under this position.

1. Standing erect, the feet 15 or 16 inches apart, interlock the hands and raise them over the head.

2. Gradually bend the body as in the second form of the "Side-lifting" position to the level of the loins. This is done in front, which is the only difference.

3. This form is also the same as the third of the "Side-lifting" position, except that it is performed thrice in front, and one breath is taken each time.

THE POSITION OF HSUEH-KUNG STANDING 薛 公

Ten forms are given under this position.

1. Open the fists, keep the fingers straight, then wind them round the ears and stop at a level with the breasts.

2. Press downwards from the breasts to the navel without stopping until the navel is reached.

3. Turn out the hands from the under part of the ribs; keep the palms directed upwards on a level with the shoulders, each hand even, 4 or

5 inches apart from the head; keep the two thumbs in front of the shoulders, the other fingers extended behind the shoulders.

4. Close the hands together, even with the underpart of the chin, the two little fingers close together with the palms upwards and the wrists and elbows close together. For the first time pronate the palms, let the two little fingers be attached, and stretch them upwards.

5. And then raise them thus over the forehead.

6. Gradually bend the fingers into the form of a hook, and form them into fists level with the chin.

7. Open the fists, the palms upwards and the thumbs close together. For the second time pronate the palms, the thumbs close together, and stretch them upwards.

8. Raise the hands over the forehead; bring the two little fingers close together; afterwards bring them down to the level of the chin, clench them into fists, then open them as before; bring the two little fingers close together and the palms directed upward over the fore-head.

9. This form is exactly related to the last. For the third time, pronate the palms, the two little fingers close together, and stretch them upwards.

10. Then lower the fingers, form them into fists, and let them be evenly and circularly arranged as if enfolding things, the two fists 18 or 19 inches apart. One breath is then taken. This is to be performed three times, so three breaths should be taken.

THE ARRANGING-ELBOW POSITION 列肘

There are three forms under this position.

1. The left foot bent, the right foot straight, the right hand is clenched and held in the left hand.

2. Stretch out the left elbow to the left and draw it back immediately; then squat with the body, the left foot straight, the other bent; let the left hand still hold the right fist, and raise the right elbow a little.

3. Raise the body, with the left foot bent and the right foot straight; lean the body to the left and take a breath; raise the right elbow higher. Perform the same on the right side—on each side three times, taking six inspirations. While the body is leaning, let the eyes look at a point six inches from the feet.

THE RESTING-ON-THE-KNEE POSITION 伏膝

The left foot bent, the right foot straight, lay the right hand on the left leg over two inches from the knee; lay the left hand on top of the right hand. Pronate the body sideways, let the face look evenly towards the left, and take a breath. With the back bowed and the neck straight, look downwards at a point more than six inches from the feet. Do the same on the right—three times on each side, and take six breaths.

THE CHAN-HSIAO POSITION 站宵

Four forms are given under this position; the first two are termed the "cannon of the den," the third the "cannon rushing against the sky," and the fourth the "cannon passing through the heart."

1. The left foot bent, the right foot straight, let the palm of the left hand face downwards level with the breast, the thumb kept inwards; let the palm of the right hand be directed upwards and level with the navel; place the little finger inwards and keep all the fingers apart.

2. Pull the hands out horizontally, then clench them; let the left one be level with the breast eight or nine inches from it, the thumb kept inwards; let the right fist be level with the ribs, over one inch from it; the thumb directed outwards, take a breath in front, then turn the head and look to the left.

3. Open the left fist and whirl it, then make it into a fist again; stretch it perpendicularly on a level with the side of the forehead. Take a breath in front and turn the head and look to the space between the thumb and second finger of the left hand.

4. Open the left fist and whirl it round the ear, then stretch the first straight out towards the left, keeping the dorsum upwards. Turn the head and look to the left, and take one breath. Do the same on the right side—on each side three times, taking altogether eighteen breaths.

THE GRAIN-BAG-BEATING POSITION 打穀袋

There are 12 forms under this position. The first two are termed "cannon rushing against the sky" 衝天礮.

1. Keep left foot bent, the right foot straight; hold the bag in the right hand, whirl the left from under the ribs, clench the fist, bend the elbow and extend it upwards; then take a breath.

2. Hold the bag with the right hand and with it beat the left arm

steadily down to the left palm and fingers several times. This is beating the inner part of the left arm.

RULE—Always beat straight down—never backwards—nor return on any omitted part. It should be done at once.

3. This is termed "cannon passing through the heart" 穿 心 礮. Open the left fist, whirl it round the ear, stretch the first straight out to the left, keeping the dorsum upwards, and take a breath. Holding the bag with the right hand, with it beat the arm steadily to the back of the hand and the tip of the middle finger. This is beating the outer part of the left arm.

4. This is termed the "vulture-hand" 雕 手 . Whirl the left hand round and take the form of a "vulture-hand;" take a breath, then hold the bag with the right hand and with it beat from the left armpit steadily down to the side of the little finger. This is beating the under part of the left upper limb.

5. This is termed the "minor cannon rushing against the sky" 小 衝 天 礮. Whirl the left hand once, then raise the fist so as to assume the form of a "cannon rushing against the sky," only a little lower, and take a breath. Now the right hand beats with the bag from the left shoulder steadily down to the side of the thumb of the left hand. This is beating the upper part of the left upper limb.

6. This and the following are both termed "carrying the tripod on the shoulder" 扛 鼎 . Whirl the left hand from under the ribs, clench the fist, stretch it straight upwards with energy, keeping the thumbs at the back part, then take a breath and look upward at the rising fist.

7. Holding the bag with the right hand, beat with it from the left ribs steadily down to the front side of the left leg, knee, shinbone, instep, and toe. This is called beating the front part of the lower left limb.

8. This is termed "coiling the elbow" 盤 肘 . Open the left fist and whirl it round the ear, then bend the elbow and clench the fist on a level with a breast; take a breath and raise the elbow a little. Now with the bag in the right hand, beat steadily from the left armpit inclined to the left loin, to the outer ankle, and to the side of the little toe. This is beating the outer part of the lower left limb.

9. This is termed the "vulture hand." Open the left fist and make a "vulture hand," and whirl it round the ear and take a breath. Then holding the bag by the right hand, beat from the end of the sternum down to the abdomen, and from the space between the ribs and abdomen beat horizontally to the right side of the abdomen; change

hands with the bag and beat horizontally to the left of the abdomen. Protect the secret parts by covering them with the right hand, and beat with the left hand beginning from the left side of the "little abdomen" steadily to the inner part of the left leg and left toe. If there is abdominal illness of any kind, it may be cured by beating several times. This is beating the inner part of the lower left limb.

10. This and the next two are called "resting-on-the-knee." The right foot bent, left foot straight, and left hand holding the bag, press on the right in the middle of the leg; also press the right hand on the bag, then take a breath.

11. Holding the bag with both hands, raise it over the head and beat the spine twenty times, but do not beat the ridge of the spine.

12. With the left foot stretched, the right foot bent, lay the right hand on the surface of the right leg; keep the thumb directed backwards, incline the body backwards, and look on the left knee. The left hand holding the bag, turn the hand back and beat the left part under the back consecutively to the loin, then return the hand and beat the left buttock, left leg, knee, and calf down to the heel. This is beating the back part of the lower left limb. After going through the exercises on the left upper and lower limbs, then transfer to the right upper and lower limbs, following the same method.

SCOOPING THE MOON AT THE BOTTOM OF THE SEA 海 底 撈 月
The position has five forms.

1. Lay the left hand on the surface of the leg and make the right into a "vulture hand," *i.e.*, bringing the tips of the fingers together.

2. Whirl the left hand round the ear and then stretch the palm out towards the left.

3. Turn the head with the back upwards.

4. In such a way as to scoop the moon, bow the head and bend the loins to scoop from left to right; then raise the body up.

5. While scooping, assume "the moon-looking" manner and take a breath, then look at the interval between the thumb and the second finger of the left hand. The same should be done on the right— thrice on each side and altogether six breaths taken.

The above 64 diagrams are the first part of the exercises, embracing 87 breaths in all.

功夫 Ta-Mo's (Bodhidharma's) Works

A work in one volume, one of the smallest, cheapest, and most popular books on Kung-fu, is the *Wei-sheng-chin-ching* 衛 生 易 筋 經, supposed by scholars to be spurious. Several abridged editions of this book are sold under the designation *Wei-sheng-yao-shu* 衛 生 要 術. The former book has a preface by Sung-Kwang-tsu 宋 光 祚 written in 1875, in which he says that:

He is a lover of good books, and he visited a great temple where Kung-fu was practised with advantage to the original air and vital spirits, not only protecting against disease but also prolonging life, and still more enabling persons to become divine sages. He had much leisure and was anxious to reprint good books, dispense medicines, and cure serious disease. People from all quarters praised his good deeds; his own evil thoughts banished, he ate and drank in an orderly way and discreetly. His one desire was to obtain peace; he had spent much time and labour in searching into prescriptions for the nourishment of the body when he came across this book, and he rejoiced to obtain the benefit of the two books *Huang-t'ing* 黃 庭 and *Nei-ching* 內 經 in learning the methods of the Immortals. He was glad to possess this book, and he wished others with the same heart as his own to reap the same advantage in helping to nourish their bodies.

This is followed by a preface written by Li Ching 李 靖, a great military officer of the T'ang dynasty, in the second year (529 A.D.) of the second Emperor of that dynasty. He says: In the time of the later Wei 後 魏, in the year T'ai-ho 太 和 of the Emperor Hsiao-ming 孝 明, the Buddhist priest Ta-mo 達 摩 [Bodhidharma—the Chinese represents the sound of the last two syllables of his Indian name] arrived at the court of Wu-ti, the first Emperor of the Liang dynasty, where he first dwelt. Afterwards he removed to the Kingdom of Wei and dwelt at a temple called Shao-lin-ssu 少 林 寺 . After a residence of nine years in China [he was sixty-nine years old when he arrived in the year 526 and was the 28th Indian patriarch], he died and was buried at the foot of Hsiung-erh Mountain 熊 耳 山 [between Honan and Shensi]. He left one shoe.

When his monument was being repaired after the course of years, an iron box, unlocked but firmly fastened with glue, was found. Upon the application of heat, the box opened. The inside was filled with wax, and it was this that rendered its opening difficult. Inside were two books, one termed the *Sui-hsi-ching* 髓 洗 經 , the other the *I-chin-ching* 易 筋 經 . The latter had to do with the conservation of the body. After generations saw nothing of the former, the latter was found at Shao-lin-ssu, written in the language of the country called T'ien-chu 天 竺 [India]. There was great difficulty in having it translated. Each one took the best meaning out of it he could and by so doing obtained the bypath—not the highway—or the leaves and branches—not the stem— and so lost the real method of becoming Immortals. At present the priests of the temple obtain advantage from the wrestling [method] merely.

One of the more intelligent argued that what Ta-mo left could not be unimportant, and so he went on a pilgrimage to Mount O-mei 峨 嵋 in Szechuan in search of one who could translate the work. There he met an Indian priest by the name of Pan-la-mi 殷 刺 密 . To him he spoke of the classic and his reason for coming. The Indian priest explained the work so far as was possible, for the language of Buddha cannot be translated; it is extraordinarily deep, deeper than water. He was invited to stay at the temple and so got initiated by degrees into the details of Kung-fu. In one hundred days he became quite strong, in one hundred more his entire body had received benefit, and after the third hundred days he was able to do everything, his constitution became as hard as steel, and he could aspire to the position of a Buddha. He accompanied the Indian priest wherever he went.

One Hsu-hung met them and obtained the secret method from them, and he gave it to a red bearded guest who gave it to the writer of the preface, who tried the method with the best results and so became a believer. He deeply regretted he did not obtain the *Sui-hsi-ching* and he also felt regrets that his convictions were not strong enough to induce him to give up all and follow the priests; not being able to carry out this plan, he felt as if there were something wanting in his heart. He complains of people not having heard of this work, and so he writes this preface to inform them how the work came into his hands, with hopes that through this they may truly learn of Buddha. That each may attain to the Kung-fu of Buddha is the ideal which Ta-mo had in his heart in bequeathing this classic. [This is an extract and the substance of the principal part of the preface.]

Ta-mo left Nanking where the Emperor resided and went to Loyang, in modern Honanfu. For nine years he sat with his face to a wall, and hence the epithet applied to him—"the wall-gazing Brahman." He died of old age. Sung Yun, who was sent in 518 A.D. to India for Buddhist books by the Prince of Wei, returned and inspected the remains of Ta-mo. As the priest lay in his coffin, he held one shoe in his hand. Sung Yun asked him whither he was going. "To the Western Heaven," was the reply. Sung then returned home. The coffin was afterwards opened and found empty; the shoe alone was lying there. This shoe was preserved as a relic in the monastery but was stolen in the T'ang dynasty.

The succeeding preface appears in the section entitled *Physiology of Kung-fu*. The concluding preface is by one Niu Kao, a military officer of the Sung dynasty, written in the twelfth year of Shao-hsing, the first Emperor of the Southern Sung (1143 A.D.).

He was an illiterate individual, he says, ignorant of written characters. He was a follower of a celebrated general named Yueh Fei 岳 飛 ; he once met a remarkable priest, so like a *lohan*.[1] In his hand he had a letter which he gave to him to give to Yueh Fei, who, he said, had divine power and was able to stretch a bow with the resistance of 100 piculs' weight; this strength was given him not by Heaven, but by the priest. "When a youth he was my pupil and he practised Kung-fu most thoroughly. I asked him to become one of my followers and adopt the doctrine of the Buddha, which, however, he said he did not believe; so he left me to the prosecute worldly affairs. He had become a great officer with a great reputation—this seems his destiny. Give him this letter and let him know the evils of the world—that he may be in Imperial favour one day and the next day in disgrace, suffering punishment; that the pursuit of the Buddhist doctrines was alone satisfying." Niu was afraid to hear the priest talk thus and asked his name, to which no reply was given.

Yueh took the letter and before finishing the perusal of it, he wept and said: "He was my master, a holy priest, and if he had not taken care of me I should have died." Thereupon he brought a book out of his

---

[1][Ed. note: The Chinese word for the Sanskrit *arhat*, a Theravada Buddhist saint.]

breast and told Niu to take it. He afterwards lost Imperial favour; in order to hand down the work, Niu Kao hid it in a wall in Sung Hill 嵩 山 , that someone hereafter finding it might propagate it, he himself being destitute of all ability. In this way he hoped to obtain some merit and be able to look Yueh Fei in the face [i.e., do something which would not only not disgrace him but in fact be a credit to him].

The work begins with the rules for Kung-fu in rhyme to be committed to memory, which we omit as their substance is embraced in the Eight Ornamental Sections. Next comes a general discourse which is also omitted. Then follows a chapter on Membranes.

There are two grand methods included in Kung-fu, the internal and the external. The internal Method has to do with the Membranes. The body is distinguished into many parts, of which the internal are the five organs, the six viscera, the animal vigour and the spirit; the external are the four limbs, the bones, sinews and flesh. These form one body. The essential parts of them are the blood and the animal vigour. To invigorate these two things are therefore of the first importance in Kung-fu.

The animal vigour and spirit are immaterial but the sinews, bones and muscles are material. The method is to discipline the material as the assistants of the immaterial and to cultivate the immaterial to aid the material. These two are intimately related. If it is desired to discipline the sinews, the animal vigour comes first in order, then the membranes, and last of all the sinews, which is then easy. To discipline the membranes is difficult, but to discipline the animal vigour is the most difficult of all. The true plan is to lay the foundation in the difficult.

The important part of Kung-fu is to nourish the original air [constitution], collect the central air, care for the perfect air, protect the kidney air, nourish the liver air, nurse the lungs, and manage the spleen, thus transforming the turbid into the pure condition, to prevent external things or emotions as grief, desire, and such-like from injuring constitution, and thus enabling it to become tranquil, pure and even; and then united, its influence will be distributed to and felt over the whole body. When it arrives at the tendons and reaches to the membranes, the entire body is then full of motion; when the air arrives at a place, the membranes rise, and when the air moves, the membranes are extended, so that the membranes and the air become equally strong.

If the sinews are disciplined and not the membranes, there is nothing for the membranes to govern, and vice versa; if the two are disciplined and not the air, the two do not increase in strength; and if vice versa, the air remains weak and fails to flow to the blood vessels. But reciprocally if the sinews are strong but are not strengthened by the air and membranes, it is like planting herbs without earth.

Pan-la-mi says that disciplining the membranes comes first, but in order to accomplish this, the discipline of the air is the lord or root of the matter. Most people do not understand the membranes. These are not the fatty membranes, but rather the membranes of the tendons; the former are inside the middle of the breast, the latter are outside the bones. The membranes are the things that connect the vessels, arms and body; they protect and are in contact with the bones and sinews of the body. Comparing the sinews and membranes, the latter are the softer; they are harder than flesh and are inside the flesh and outside the bones; they are the substances that embrace the bone and support the flesh. In Kung-fu the air must traverse to the middle of the membranes, protect the bones, and strengthen and support the sinews, which together form one body. This is the whole of Kung-fu.

The discourse on internal vigour embraces three laws. First is protecting the animal vigour, which includes attention to the five senses and motives. The best way to begin is by kneading, at which time the clothes are to be opened and the recumbent position adopted, with one palm placed on the space between the chest and abdomen. This is what is termed the "medium" where the animal vigour is stored, and it must be protected by closing the eyes and ears, equalizing the breath of the nose, shutting up the breath of the mouth, not overtoiling the strength of the body, and preventing desire and evil thoughts. This is thinking of the "middle," and the road is then well-regulated simply because the animal vigour, the essence, and the spirit are accumulated here.

Second is the absence of thought. The animal vigour, the essence and spirit, and also the blood are not independent, but are under the control of motives and follow what the motives originate. It is necessary for the motives to agree with the palm [of the hand] when protecting the "medium;" if the motive should jump to another part of the body, the vigour, essence and spirit will be scattered, and then it will become external rather than internal vigour.

Third is the management of a sufficient circulation. The kneading and guarding have for their object the prevention of the dissipation of the air which has already been collected into one place; the animal vigour, the essence and the blood will follow. By thus watching over it, we keep it from escaping; kneading it for a long time, the vigour is stored in the "medium" and prevented from running over to other parts of the body. Vigour being so accumulated, energy will also accumulate, and when the vigour is sufficient, then the energy will circulate. This air is what Mencius had in view when he said that the greatest and strongest is the strength of air, which can fill the entire heaven and earth [i.e., air without limit]. If the air is not full and has not circulated, and the motives are scattered, it is not only internal but also external robustness that is devoid of strength.

Pan-la-mi held with Mencius that human nature was originally good, that the good was gradually covered by the evil which found admission through the senses—the body and ideas—and clouded the understanding, so that a partition, as it were, has come in between the individual and the Doctrine (*Tao*). So Ta-mo at Shao-lin-ssu remained nine years ignorant of mundane affairs, and by shutting the eye and ear was able to tie, as it were, his ideas, which are like the monkey or the horse, so fleet that one cannot catch them; and so the *Tao* is closed, but shutting up the senses is like binding these two animals. So Ta-mo secured the true method and left a shoe and went to the West [died] and thus became one of the Immortals. Ta-mo left this true method and the *Shou-chung* (the shutting out of the world and guarding the "medium," thus preventing its dissipation). In this way an ignorant person can become wise and a weak one strong, and so arrive quickly at the Happy Land.

The drugs recommend for internal robustness are the following [Ed.: a rare prescription]: Take of *Yeh-chi-li* 野 蒺 藜, Tribulus terrestris (roasted and the seeds removed); *pai-fu-ling* (skin removed); *pai-shuo-tao* (roasted a little with wine); *shou-ti-huang* (prepared with wine); licorice (made with honey); *chu-sha* (vermillion, precipitated with water) —of each 5 ounces; ginseng; *pai-shu* (roasted with earth); *tang-kuei (prepared with wine)*; *ch'uaen-hsiung*—of each 1 ounce. Powder and, with honey, make into pills of 1 mace in weight. Dose: 1 to be swallowed with soup or wine.

It is said that with pills made up of so many ingredients, the strength is not unified but must vary and go into different channels; so three prescriptions are added, any one of which may be taken.

(1) Take *chi-li* deprived of its pricks and make into pills with honey; take 1 or 2 mace. [This plant is of extreme value, it is said, in bringing donkeys rapidly into fine condition.]

(2) *Chu-sha*, 3 candareens, washed in water. Swallow in honey water.

(3) *Fu-ling*, skin removed. Powder and make into pills with honey, or mix with water and so take, or make into a paste and dissolve in honey water.

KNEADING

The idea of kneading is rubbing or shampooing the sinews and bones strong. It consists of three portions, each of one hundred days.

1. Kneading in Season

If one begins in spring when the weather is still a little cold and the body is closely wrapped up in clothes, it is only necessary to open the upper clothes. In the middle of the second month when the weather has grown warmer, the lower part of the body may then be exercised, and thereafter one may practise most conveniently.

2. Certain Forms of Kneading

The animal vigour [air] is situated on the right side of the body, and the blood on the left. In kneading one must begin and advance from the right to the left. The *raisons d'etre* are three. To push the vigour so that it enters the blood and makes them mix. To broaden the stomach so that it may receive more vigour. The stomach is situated on the right side. The right palm of the kneader is more powerful than the left.

3. The Quality of the Kneading

It must be light and superficial. The process, although the individual's, ought to be in accordance with heaven's laws and with the production of things by heaven and earth—that is, slowly, little by little and not suddenly. When the air arrives it necessarily causes growth; then wait till it is complete. Kneading ought to be done after this fashion; the pushing ought to be even and uniform, slowly coming and going backwards and forwards, not too heavy and not too deep. When one has exercised for a long time, then one obtains the advantages; this is the proper thing. If [the kneading is] too heavy, the skin may be injured and disease perhaps set up [such as pityriasis versicolor and lichen tropicus]; if it is too deep, the muscles, sinews and membranes may inflame and swell. Hence the necessity of care.

In refining the animal vigour by external exercises we use kneading, and at the time of practising the exercise, a medicine pill is taken. When it is conjectured that the pill is dissolved [in the stomach], use the kneading; the strength of the pill unites with the kneading and thus the advantage is obtained. No benefit accrues from beginning the kneading before the pill has dissolved nor long after it has dissolved. Knead and take a pill once in three days and continue in this manner. [The ingredients of the pills have been already given].

Another matter to be attended to under Kung-fu is constantly washing and bathing the body in brine. The salted water can make the hard soft and disperse the heat. It is performed daily or once in two days. The prescription is to take of the root-bark of Lycium Chinense and salt, of each *ad libitum*, in warm water; thus the blood and air will harmonize and the skin and epidermis will feel most comfortable.

The third thing calling for attention is the wooden pestle and mallet, both of which are made of hard wood. The pestle is 6 inches long, the mid part ½ inch in diameter, the head round, and the tail sharp (a knob at one end and a point at the other end). The mallet is 1 foot long, 4 inches in circumference; the handle is slender at the upper part, the top is thick with a knob at the end, and at the middle of the body is a little higher. (See illustrations)

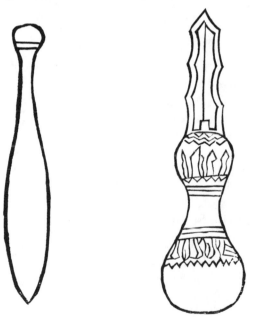

The fourth thing is the pebble bag. It is necessary to beat the muscles with the wooden pestle and mallet, but the joints must be exercised with the pebble bag. It is made of linen cloth, in form not unlike the pestle and of three different sizes, the major one 8 inches long and 1 catty in weight, the medium one 6 inches long and 12 ounces in weight, and the minor one 5 inches long and ½ catty in weight. The size of the largest pebbles must not exceed the size of the grape, and of the smaller the pomegranate seed, and only those must be used which have been found in water and are free from edges and corners.

1. Kung-fu for the First Month

At the beginning of kneading, a succession of little boys is required, for they possess little strength and so knead not so heavily, and their animal vigour is strong. First swallow the pill, and just as it begins to be digested commence the kneading; the advantage is to be gained when the two go hand in hand. At the beginning of the kneading, the dress on the breast must be opened. Recline and place the palm of the hand on the part below the heart and above the navel, and knead from the right to the left, slowly coming and going, not so light that the hand leaves the skin and not so heavy as to press heavily upon the bones, and not performed confusedly. This is the proper mode. While kneading, the heart must look inwards [*i.e.*, denuded of all external thought], the idea guarded in the "medium," and the thoughts not allowed to roam outside; thus the essence, the air and the spirit are all below the palm. This is truly the golden mean (*huo hou* 火 候).

At this period there is no scattering of the thoughts, and the kneading is equalized. If this condition is attained, one can sleep during the process and the method is all the more remarkable; the *shou-ching* idea is better when the person is asleep. The duration of the exercise must be about the time taken to burn two sticks of incense, three time each day, morning, noon and evening. If the person is young and strong, twice daily, morning and evening, will be sufficient; if more frequently performed harm might be the result. After kneading, a short sleep is advisable, after which other business may be engaged in without detriment.

2. Kung-fu for the Second Month

The animal vigour has accumulated during the first month, the stomach has become large and broad, and the sinews on the sides of the abdomen have been raised over 1 inch and can, when pressed with air, become as hard as wood or stone. This is the result. But the space between the sinews from the heart to the navel is still soft and hollow, because the membranes are deeper than the sinews and the palm kneading has not yet reached them; consequently they have not risen.

This time, knead by the side of the palm so as to open [another] palm according to the former method, and pound deeply the soft parts with the wooden pestle; after a time the membranes will be raised above the skin and possess the same strength as the sinews, without being either soft or hollow. This is the complete *kung*. The period occupied by kneading and pounding must be that of two sticks of incense thrice daily, and by the use of this exercise daily no defect will be developed.

3. Kung-fu for the Third Month

After two months' exercise, the hollow space in the centre is a little raised; then gently beat with the wooden mallet on the kneaded portion of the two sides of the first palm "width," and pound with the wooden pestle the parts which reach the end of the two great sinews 1 "palm wide," according to the kneading method. The time occupied is to equal the time taken in burning two sticks of incense, thrice daily.

4. Kung-fu for the Fourth Month

Three months' exercise being now completed, the three middle "palm-wide" parts are all beaten by the wooden mallet, and the external two "palm-wide" parts are first pounded, then beaten, thrice daily, each for a period equal to the burning of two sticks of incense. After exercising over one hundred days, the air becomes full, the sinews strong, and the membranes raised; thus advantage is reaped.

5. Light and Heavy Method of Performing the Kung

In beginning the exercise, light manipulation is of the first importance, and a young boy must be employed because his strength is even; after one month when the air has slowly increased, the strength can be increased. It must not be used too strongly in case inflammation should be set up; it must be pursued in strict order and not confusedly, in case the skin should get injured. Therefore care must be exercised.

6. Deep and Superficial Method of Performing the Kung

In the beginning the exercise is superficial; the strength increases daily, because the air is becoming stronger and therefore the weight may be gradually increased, although it is still superficial. Following this, the pestle is used to pound, which can be done deeply. Afterwards beat, and although the beating outside is shallow, the movement is felt deeply inside; this is to make both the inside and outside strong, and in this way benefit accrues.

7. Internal and External Kung-fu for the Ribs

The animal vigour is full when the *kung* have been performed over one hundred days, like a mountain torrent which is full to the brim, and there is no place to which it cannot flow if a channel is left for it. At this time, therefore, precautions must be adopted to keep the air from escaping to the four extremities through improper pounding or beating outside the kneaded position; otherwise, if there is the slightest idea of conducting it elsewhere, it will become external strength [robustness]. If once the animal vigour has thus become external, it cannot be brought back and made to enter the bones, and so it cannot become internal robustness.

In order to make it enter inside, the pebble bag already described is used. Beginning at the "mouth of the heart" [breast] and proceeding to the end of the ribs, the space between the bones and muscles must be closely pounded, again kneading and beating them. After a long time the animal vigour which has accumulated will be led to the bones and will not overflow to the limbs. This is internal robustness.

Here the distinction between inside and outside is to be observed and maintained; if not clearly differentiated in such actions as drawing the two, moving the fists, beating or grasping a thing, the air will proceed to the outside and can never be brought back to the inside, so it is necessary to use the utmost care.

8. Kung-fu for the Fifth, Sixth, Seventh and Eighth Months

The exercises on the ribs have not been performed for over one hundred days, and we have already beaten with the pebble bag and kneaded from below the "mouth of the heart" to the end of the ribs on the two sides—that is, the part where the clefts of the bones unite, and where the external and internal robustness divide. If at this place it is undesirable to lead the vigour to the outside, the accumulated air can enter the fissures of the bones, following the course of the beating.

One ought to beat from the breast to the neck and from the ends of the ribs to the shoulder, performing revolution after revolution in this manner but never retrograding, thrice daily, occupying the time taken to burn six sticks of incense. This *kung* must be done continuously and without intermission for one hundred days, until the breast in front becomes full, and the *Fen* pulse is also full. The Kung-fu is now half finished.

9. Kung-fu for the Ninth, Tenth, Eleventh and Twelfth Months

When the Kung-fu has been performed for two hundred days, the animal vigour in the front of the chest is full and the *Fen* pulse full, the vigour must be transferred to the back and made to communicate with the *Tu* pulse.

The air has already reached to the shoulder and neck. The former method must be pursued in beating and kneading, going upwards to the occiput, in the middle of the spine between the scapulae, and downwards to the coccyx, beating each part, returning, repeating the operation and never retrograding. The soft parts on the sides of the spine must be kneaded with the palm or pounded and beaten by the pestle and mallet thrice daily, occupying the time taken to burn six sticks of incense, whether above or below, right or left kneading or beating one revolution. In this way in one hundred days the back will be full of air, dissipating all manner of disease, and the *Tu* pulse full to overflowing. After each beating it must be rubbed with the hand in order to make it uniform.

[Ed.: Severael sections were omitted here due to their subject matter, which is related to sex.] One is entitled the Method of Pairing the Yin and Yang Principles. Another is called the Method for Applying Kung-fu to the Lower Portion of the Body. A third is termed Things Forbidden in the Practice of Kung-fu.

Then follows a Prescription for the Washing of the Lower Portion of the Body, the object of which is to cause the efficacy of the drugs to be communicated to the air and unite with the blood in the system, to toughen the skin, to dissipate the heat, and to free the system from desire. The receipt is as follows: Take of *she-ch'uang-tzu,* 蛇 床 子 Selinum Monnieri; root bark of Lycium Chinense; and licorice *ad libitum*. Make a decoction, fomenting the parts once or twice daily.

JOINING BATTLE

1. Internal Robustness and "Divine Strength"

We have not yet exhausted the subject of internal and external energy, so we must now exhibit it. Since we have used the *kung* by beating and kneading the ribs, the air has reached to the joints, the two pulses *Fen* and *Tu* have become full, the air has circulated and filled everywhere, and before and behind have entered into communication; still we have not yet perceived any great addition of strength. How then do we speak of strength (energy), because the air (energy) has not yet reached to the hands?

The method for securing this is by the use of the pebble bag already described, beginning with the right shoulder and beating bit by bit down to the back of the middle finger; then from the back of the shoulder beating down to the back of the thumb and forefinger; then again from the front of the shoulders beating down to the back of the ring and little fingers; once more from the inside of the shoulder beating to the palm and the end of the thumb and forefinger; and again from the outside of the shoulder beating to the palms and ends of the middle and little fingers. When the beating is finished, the hand must rub and knead to make them uniform. Thrice daily—time, six sticks of incense. Also, frequently wash with warm water in order to cause the blood and air to flow together. After thus exercising one hundred days, the air has reached to all parts.

The same exercises must be gone through with the left hand for the same length of time, and then by this time "divine strength" is developed in the inside of the bones. In the course of time, go on adding exercise after exercise; the arm, the wrist, fingers and palm will become totally different from what they were formerly. Then, taking hold of the idea and using energy, they will become as hard as stone and iron, the fingers will be able to go through a bullock's abdomen, and the palm on edge will be able to decapitate a bullock's head. This is but a very small particle of the benefit to be derived from Kung-fu.

2. Exercise in order to Transport Superfluous Strength to the Hands

The plan to be adopted is to constantly bathe the hands in warm water —at first warm, then hot, then very hot. Both palm and wrists should be washed, and after washing they should not be thoroughly dried, but shaken and so dried spontaneously. While washing the hands in this way, use force to press the air in order to make it reach to the points of the fingers. This is the method for producing strength. Then fill a vessel with mixed black and green peas and constantly dip the hands into the vessel.

The bathing and washing above mentioned was with the object of harmonizing the blood and air; the object of the two sorts of peas is to disperse and remove the "fire" poison; and the dipping is to strengthen the skin by rubbing it. By using this sort of Kung-fu for a long time, the accumulated air can be forwarded to the hand and the strength thus become complete; the skin, sinews and membranes will mutually be strengthened and closely embrace the bones, neither soft nor hard. If this is not used, it will be as with ordinary mortals, but if it is used and the idea exercised, it will become as strong as iron and stone, and nothing will be able to withstand it.

This strength is developed from the bones and is totally different from what is usually termed external robustness. The difference between outside and inside robustness is to be recognized by the sinews. In the internal, the sinews are long and comfortable, the skin is fine and glossy and the strength is heavy [intense]; in the external, the skin is coarse and tough, the various sinews of the palms and wrists are coiled like the common earthworm and apparent on the skin, and the strength, although great, has no root. This is the difference between the two.

3. The External Robustness and Divine Strength of the Eight Ornamental Sections

After one has obtained internal robustness and the firm consolidation of the strength of the bones, it can then be led to the outside, because the inside has a root and it can be driven to the outside, and so become the root of the science. In disciplining the outside *kung*, there are the eight methods: lifting, holding up, pushing, pulling, clutching, pressing, seizing, and overflowing.

Perform these eight methods energetically, each method once; repeat times without number, thrice daily about the time that six sticks of incense would take to burn. After a long time when the *kung* is finished the whole body will be filled with strength. When required, it will be freely developed without fail. When people hear of this they are thunderstruck.

The ancients thought that lifting the portcullis was a feat of marvellous strength [referring to a Herculean feat of this sort performed by K'ung-shu-liang-ho, the father of Confucius, who was renowned for his great personal prowess and unusual strength], and they admired the strength capable of lifting a tripod [referring to Wu Yun and Pa Wang, who could lift a tripod 1000 catties in weight, the latter being the Hercules or Samson of China]. Practise the above eight methods separately one after the other and the greatest benefit is to be derived therefrom; if otherwise minded, follow the exercise *sua volonte*.

4. Added Kung to the Divine Strength

Internal and external *kung*, being now both complete, can be termed Divine Strength; although complete, it must afterwards be constantly employed and not thrown aside at will. You must find growing out in the garden a large tree, which obtains the air of the soil and wood, which causes it to grow, and which is different from that of other localities. When you have leisure you must proceed to the shade of the tree, and, according to your own convenience, practise the exercises—whether beating, rubbing, pushing, drawing, kicking or pulling up—in order to obtain the growing energy of the tree to produce or excite your vitality; during leisure you can complete the *kung-fu*.

Again, search out a wilderness adjoining hills, and find a large erect stone that has grown beautiful and is the finest to be found. Constantly resort to it, practise pushing, pressing and the other above-mentioned exercises, and obtain the auspiciousness of the site; if you can obtain this air, there is certainly great advantage. In ancient times the Great Shun dwelt beside stones and wood, and his practise was not devoid of meaning.

These are followed by the Twelve Ornamental Sections, which are simply an amplification of the Eight already given. They are derived from the Buddhist sect, in which meditation is the important thing.

If one proposes to practise these exercises, the first thing is to close the eyes, shut the heart, and close the hands tightly. All worldly affairs are to be banished, the heart must be perfectly pure and the breath harmonized, and then the spirit will be fixed; afterwards perform the *kung* according to the order and forms given, and the energy and idea will react to the place desired. The exercise of the form without the idea is useless; if the heart as governor wanders here and there and the spirit and idea are both dissipated, the trouble of the exercise is borne in vain; no good is to be derived from the *kung*. At first, in disciplining the movements, the heart and strength must both have arrived [at the place desired in the exercise]; this is the movement, the peaceful repose, the heart thinking of the number thirty times, and daily increasing up to one hundred times. Perform this thrice daily, and after twenty days the *kung* are complete. When the air and strength are obtained, thrice daily will do, and when the air and strength are strongly consolidated, once daily will do. The important thing in all these exercises is that the idea constantly accompanies them.

THE EIGHTEEN DISCIPLINARY RECORDS

1. The Method of Rubbing the Shoulder and Wrist

On the completion of the *kung*, first stretch out the left arm and let another lift up the "tiger's mouth" [the space between the thumb and forefinger] with both hands. Rub energetically and gradually increase the times; if at first it was ten times, increase gradually to one hundred times. The right arm is to be rubbed in the same manner. The object aimed at is to produce heat in the two shoulders and wrists which will reach to the bones.

2. Disciplinary Beating of the Hands and Feet

At first, according to one's strength, have a cloth bag made of two layers in which are five or six catties of small gravel or sand; hang it on a frame. In performing the *kung*, constantly push it with the palm, beat it with the fist, kick it and step upon it with the feet. The important thing is to keep the bag in motion, pushing and kicking it back. As time goes on, gradually increase the weight of the sand in the bag.

3. The Method of Disciplining the Fingers

One must calculate one's own strength—whether it is great or small—and select a round, smooth, clean stone of one or two catties in weight. Grasp it with five fingers, let it go, and again seize it before it reaches the ground. At first practise this several times, and after a while regularly increase the number of times and the weight of the stone. Thus the five fingers will become strong.

Another method is: When sitting at any time, press the seat with the fingers and gently raise the body. In this way the fingers themselves will develop strength. This exercise can be done whether one or many are present, and after a time the result will be evident.

This is followed by a section on the "Jade Ring" Aperture; and this again by prescriptions entitled the Elixir Capable of Beating a Tiger, the Great Strength Pills, the Immortals' Receipt for Washing the Hands and for Strengthening the Sinews and Bones. The two pulses, the *Fen* (running down the middle of the body in front) and *Tu* (from the vertex to the coccyx), and the acupuncture apertures are next described. Then follows a chapter on the number of bones in the body; next on the blood vessels; then a discourse on the air and blood, the former being taken in the old sense of our artery, and the latter being the veins, or only real blood vessels—in this case a most convincing proof of the knowledge of the blood's circulation possessed by the Chinese. [Ed.: All are very important chapters and will be dealt with in a future book.]

METHOD FOR ACQUIRING THE ESSENCES OF THE SUN AND MOON

[The important thing is to have the lungs full of air.] The two essences of the Sun and Moon must unite to produce the myriad things of nature. The ancients swallowed these essences and in time became Immortals. The method is secret. People in the world are ignorant of it.

Even among those who know it, if their will is not strong and with want of constant practice, it becomes useless. Although those who daily exercise the *kung* are few, if it is done from the beginning and continued until it is complete and until death, whether one is at leisure or busy and whether or not one has any outside business—if only it is done daily and constantly, one can become an immortal without much difficulty. By receiving and swallowing it, the essence of the sun and moon is added to the spirit and intelligence, and then ignorance and all crudities are dissolved, the person feels full of vigour and is very efficient, and the myriad diseases are not developed. Truly the benefit is great.

The method is that daily on the first of the month (*shuo*), when the air is new and fresh, and during the last half (*wang*) when metal and water (two of the Five Elements) are full and the air is perfect and progressive, at this time one can obtain the lunar essence. If it rains or is cloudy on any of these days, or if one lacks leisure on those days, the 2nd, 3rd, 16th and 17th will also do, and so can also increase the vigour and essence; after these six days, when the sun is inclining to the West and the moon becomes smaller and weaker, their essence is insufficient and therefore unimportant to health.

In speaking of the sun, its essence ought to be swallowed on the 1st and 15th between 3 and 7 A.M. One must go to a high place opposite the sun, remain perfectly still, harmonize the air inspired by the nose and slowly inhale one full mouthful of the solar essence; then close the respiration, collect the animal vigour, and slowly swallow it little by little while thinking; let the idea introduce it into the Central Palace [the *tan-t'ien*]. This is the manner of performing one act of deglutition, and it must be repeated seven times. Then stop a little, retaining it, after which you may repair home and attend to your ordinary business without inconvenience. [Perform this also] during the lunar diminution [the sun and moon are said to be full on the 1st and 15th respectively] according to the foregoing method, from 7 to 11 P.M., also seven times repeated.

This is the principle pervading heaven and earth. If one pursues it with a constant and fixed heart, great advantage can be obtained; those who believe it can lay hold of it and use it. This is the method for performing a very large and important *kung*. Do not reckon it unimportant and make no mistake in regard to it.

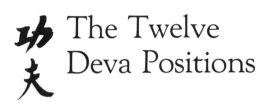 The Twelve
Deva Positions

1. The First Aspect of Wei-to Offering the Pestle.

Stand upright and form a ring with the hands.
Apply them to the heart.
Fix the breath and gather in the spirit (energy), with a pure heart and
respectful countenance.

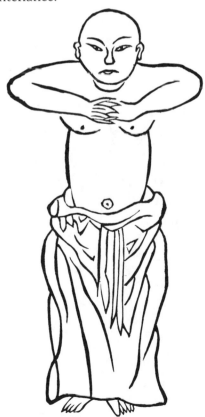

2. The Second Aspect of Wei-to[1]

Apply the toes to the ground.
Stretch out the arms horizontally, with quieted heart and silent breath.
Fix the eyes wide open and mouth simple.

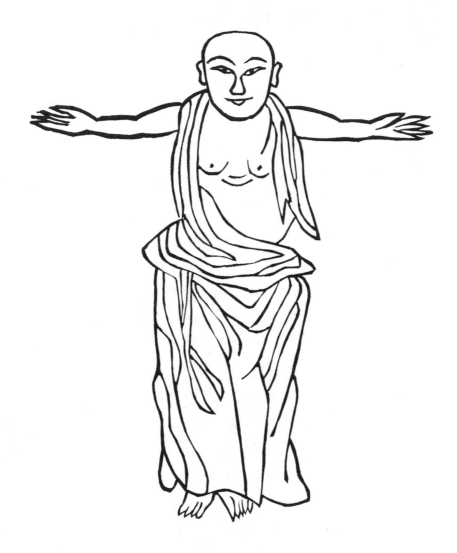

[1]A *deva* or inhabitant of heaven, who protects the Buddhist religion and three of the four continents into which the world is divided. It is the name of the Bodhisattva general under the Four Great Kings, who stands in the front hall of all Buddhist monasteries.

3. The Third Aspect of Wei-to

Support Heaven's door with the palms and look upward.
Fix the toes on the ground and stand upright.
Let energy circulate to the legs and ribs, to make them stand firm.
Close the jaws firmly and do not let them loose.
The tongue can produce saliva if it reaches the palate.
The heart will have peace if the breath is equalized by the nose.
Let the two fists gradually return to their original place.
Exert the strength as if about to carry heavy objects.

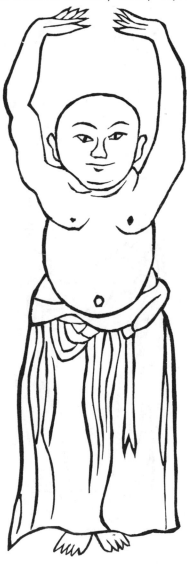

4. Taking Away a Star and Changing the Dipper for It

Support heaven and cover the head with one hand.
Fix the eyes and look through the palms.
Exert strength and turn back, on each side alike.

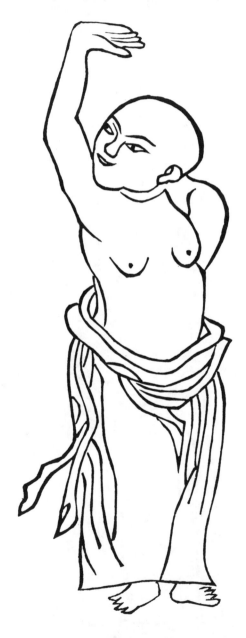

5. Pulling Nine Oxen's Tails Backwards

Stretch one leg backward, bend the other forward.
Let the small abdomen [below the navel] loosely revolve the breath.
Exert power in the two shoulders.
Fix the eyes on the fist.

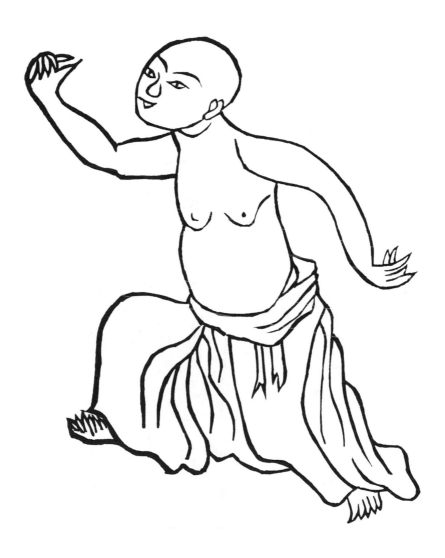

6. Pushing out the Claws and Extending the Wings

Fix the body and let the eyes be angry.
Push the hands forward in front of the chest.
With strength turn back
Seven times to complete the exercise.

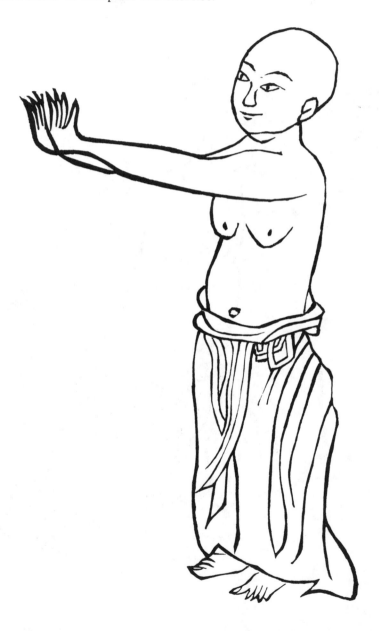

7. Nine Devils Drawing a Dagger

Half turn the head and bend the arms.
Enfold the vertex and the cervix.
When turning back from the head,
Don't object that the force is terrible.
Set in alternate rotation,
With body upright and pure breath.

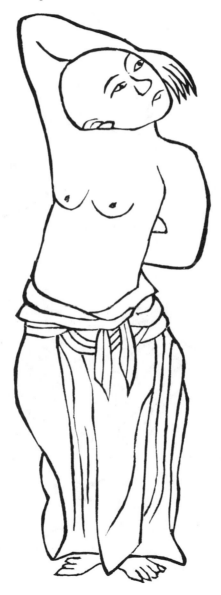

8. Three Plates Falling on the Ground

The tongue firmly attached to the palate,
Open the eyes and fix the breath.
Standing with open feet in squatting form,
The hands press forcibly as if seizing something.
Turn the palms at the same time,
A weight seeming more than a thousand catties.
Open the eyes and shut the mouth.
Stand upright, the feet not aslant.

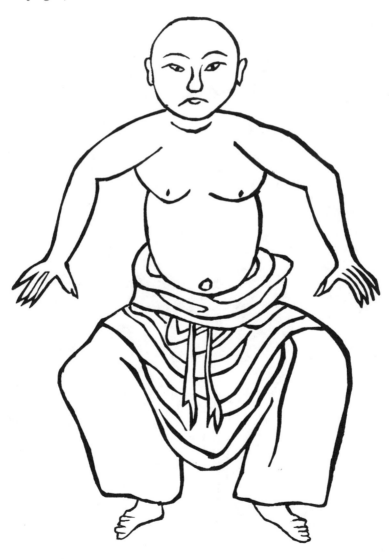

9. The Azure Dragon Stretching Its Claws

The Azure Dragon stretches its claws.
The left emerges from the right.
The exercise imitates it.
Level the palms and deeply breathe.
Exert strength on the shoulders and back.
Circling around, pass the knee.
Fix the eyes on the level.
The breath is equalized, and the heart quiet.

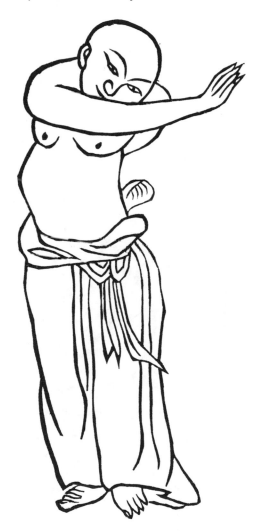

10. The Lying Tiger Springing at His Food

Stand with the feet apart as if the body would upset.
Bend and stretch each leg alternately.
Raise up the head that the breast may stretch forward.
Flatten the back and let the loins be level as a flat smooth stone.
Equalize the in-and-out-going breath by the nose.
Let the tips of the fingers rest on the ground and raise the body.
To vanquish the dragon and reduce the tiger [*i.e.*, the influence of the
    Immortals],
Learn to obtain a true body and so protect one's health.

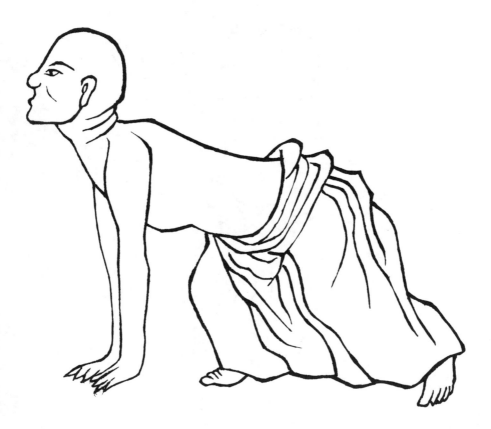

11. Making a Bow

Hold the head by the hands.
Bend the waist to between the knees.
Stretch the head to between the legs.
Close the jaws very tightly.
Cover up the ears to the sense of hearing as if something were inserted
    in them.
Arrange the original air in a restful condition.
Attach the tip of the tongue firmly to the palate.
Exert force at the bending elbow.

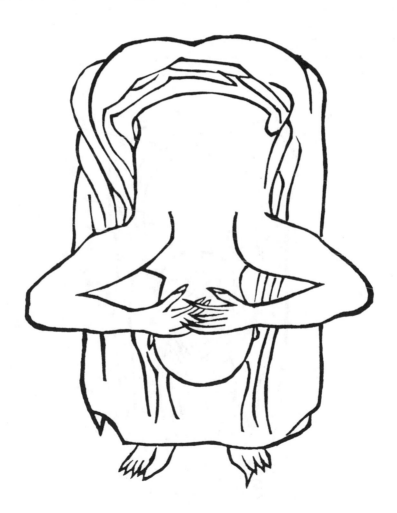

12. Wagging the Tail

With upright legs and outstretched arms,
Push the hands to the ground.
Fix the eyes and raise the head.
Settle the thoughts and think of nothing else.
Raise the head and feet.
One and twenty times,
On each side stretch the arms.
Take seven as the limit,
Still more to perform the sitting *kung*.
Bend one leg under the other and hang the eyelids down.
Fix the mouth to the heart.
Equalize the breath by the nose.
When one has entered the state of quietism, then arise.
The exercise is then complete.

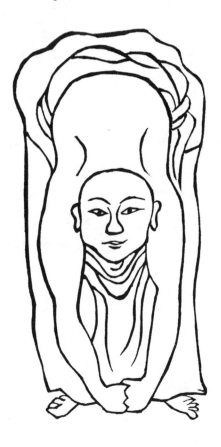

Examine these methods.
There are twelve illustrations.
From the time of the Five Kingdoms,
Whom has really learned this method?
Ta-mo came from the West,
And spread the doctrines at Shao-lin-ssu.
In Sung there was Yueh-hou
As an example.
To cure disease and lengthen life's span,
These exercises are unique and imcomparable.

Appendix A
MEDICINAL HERB INDEX

柴胡	Ch'ai-hu	Bupleurum falcatum
菖蒲	Ch'ang-p'u	Acorus calamus
陳皮	Ch'en-p'i	Orange peel
姜黃	Chiang-huang	Curcuma longa (turmeric)
羌活	Ch'iang-huo	Peucedanum decursivum
桔梗	Chieh-keng	Platycordon grandiflorum
建蔻仁	Chien-k'ou-jen	Nutmeg kernels from Fukien
枳殼	Chih-ch'io (or Chih-k'o)	Aegle sepiaria
赤茯苓	Ch'ih-fu-ling	Red variety of Fu-ling (See)
知母	Chih mu	Anemmorrhena asphodeloides
赤芍	Ch'ih-shao	Paeonia albiflora (cultivated variety which bears red flowers)
枳實	Chih-shih	Small fruit of Aegle sepiaria
	Chih-so	See So-sha-mi
梔子	Chih-tzu	Gardenia florida
金鈴子	Chin-ling-tzu	Fruit of Melia japonica
金銀花	Chin-yin-hua	Lonicera japonica
荊芥	Ching-chieh	Salvia plebeia
荊芥穗	Ching-chieh-sui	See Ching-chieh
青皮	Ch'ing-p'i	Immature fruits of species of citrus
橘核仁	Chu-ho-jen	Orange seed kernels
猪苓	Chu-ling	Tuberiform bodies of unknown nature
竹葉	Chu-yeh	Bamboo leaves
川芎	Ch'uan-hsiung	Pleurospermum Sp. or Conioselinum univitatum (umbelliferae)
川續斷	Ch'uan-hsu-tuan	Dipsacus asper of Lamium album from Szechuan
川牛膝	Ch'uan-niu-hsi	See Niu-hsi
川獨活	Ch'uan-tu-huo	See Tu-huo

防巳	Fang-chi	Roots and bulbs (?)
防風	Fang-feng	Peucedanum terebinthaceum? (root of an umbellifera)
茯苓	Fu-ling	Fungoid growths on roots of Pachyma cocos
茯苓皮	Fu-ling-p'i	See Fu-ling
伏神	Fu-shen	
海桐皮	Hai-t'ung-p'i	Acanthopanax ricinifolium or Bombax malabaricum
厚朴	Hou-p'o	Flowers of Szechuan hou-p'o-tzu
細辛	Hsi-hsin	Asarum Sieboldi
香附	Hsiang-fu	Cyperus rotundus
辛夷	Hsin-i	Buds of Magnolia conspicua (or M. Kobus)
玄胡索	Hsuan-hu-so	Tubers of Corydalis ambigua
滑石	Hua-shih	Talc
黃芪	Huang-ch'i	Astragalus
黃芩	Huang-ch'in	Scutellaria viscidula
黃連	Huang-lien	Rhizome of Coptis teeta
黃柏	Huang-po	Phellodendron amurense or Pterocarpus flavus
茴香	Hui-hsiang	Foeniculum vulgaris (fennel)
霍香	Huo-hsiang	Lophantus rugosus (bishopwort)
薏苡仁	I-i-jen	Seeds of Coix lachryma
人参	Jen-shen	Root of Aralia quinquefolia (pansax Ginseng)
甘菊花	Kan-chu-hua	Chrysanthemum sinense (sweet)
乾葛	Kan-ko	Pachyrhizus angulatus
藁本	Kao-pen	Nothosmyrnium japonicum
梗葉	Keng-yeh	Hemiptelea Davidi (Zelkora Davidi)
葛根	Ko-ken	Pachyrhisus angulatus
枸杞子	Kou-ch'i-tzu	Lycium chinense
故紙	Ku-chih	Legumes of Psoralea (Bauchee seeds)
苦参	K'u-shen	Root of Sophora flavescens or gustifolia
桂枝	Kuei-chih	Bark of cassia twigs
歸身	Kuei-shen	See Tang-kuei
荔枝核	Li-chih-ho	Stones of Nephelium Lichti (lichee)
良薑	Liang-chiang	Alpinia officinarum (Galangal)

連翹		Lien-ch'iao	Valves of the fruit of Forsythia suspensa
蓮鬚		Lien-hsu	See Lien-jui
蓮蕊		Lien-jui	Stamens of lotus flowers
蘿葡子		Lo-fu-tzu	Raphanus sativus (radish seeds)
綠礬		Lu-fan	Green alum (sulphate of iron?)
龍膽草		Lung-tan-ts'ao	Gentiana scabra
麻黃		Ma-huang	Ephedra vulgaris
麥冬		Mai-tung	Tubers of Ophiopogon japonicus
麥芽		Mai-ya	Sprouts of wheat and barley
蔓荊子		Man-ching-tzu	A kind of turnip with a white tuber below ground
牡桂		Mou-kuei	Cinnamomum cassia
木香		Mu-hsiang	Root of Aplotaxis auriculata (putchuck)
木瓜		Mu-kua	Pyrus Cathayensis (Chinese quince)
木賊		Mu-tsei	Equisetum japonicum
木通		Mu-t'ung	Clematis
南星		Nan-hsing	Arisaema japonicum (?)
牛膝		Niu-hsi	Achyrranthes bidentata, var. japonica
莪朮		O-shu	Kampferia pandurata
白殭蠶		Pai-chiang-ts'an	
白芷		Pai-chih	Root of Angelica anomala
白附子		Pai-fu-tzu	Arisaema sp.
白芍		Pai-shao	Paeonia albiflora
白朮		Pai-shu	Atractylis lancea var. ovata formalyrata
半夏		Pan-hsia	Tubers of Pinellia tuberifera (or rad. Ari macrori)
檳榔		Pin-lang	Areca catechu (betel-nut)
蒲黃		P'u-huang	Typha sp.
補骨脂		Pu-ku-chih	Psoralea corylifolia
桑白皮		Sang-pai-p'i	Root bark of Morus alba (mulberry)
砂仁		Sha-jen	Cardamoms
沙苑蒺藜		Sha-yuan-chi-li	Seeds of unknown plant
山茶		Shan-cha (Shan-ch'a?)	Camellia reticulata?
山查肉		Shan-ch'a-jou	Fruit of Crataegus pinnatifida
山茱萸		Shan-chu-yü	Fruit of shrub not yet identified
山藥		Shan-yao	Dioscorea Sp. (yams)
稍烏蛇肉		Shao-wu-she-jou	Flesh of small matrix pryeri (?)

芍藥	*Shao-yao*	See *Pai-shao*
神麴	*Shen-ch'u*	Medicine cake for curing colds and dispersing wind
升麻	*Sheng-ma*	Astilbe chinensis
生地	*Sheng-ti*	Rehmannia glutinosa
石菖蒲	*Shih-ch'ang-p'u*	Acorus gramineus
熟地	*Shu-ti*	See *Sheng-ti*
縮砂莔	*So-sha-mi*	Amomum villosum
蘇梗	*Su-keng*	Perilla ocymoides
酸棗仁	*Suan-tsao-jen*	Seeds of Diospyros lotus
大腹	*Ta-fu*	Betel-nut skin
大腹皮	*Ta-fu-p'i*	See *Ta-fu*
大茴香	*Ta-hui-hsiang*	See *Hui-hsiang*
丹皮	*Tan-p'i*	Root bark of Paeonia montan
當歸	*Tang-kuei*	Ligusticum acutilobum
地骨皮	*Ti-ku-p'i*	Root bark of Lycium chinense
天花粉	*T'ien-hua-fen*	Root of Trichosanthes multiloba
天麻	*T'ien-ma*	Gastrodia elata
丁香	*Ting-hsiang*	Flower buds of Eugenia carophyllata (cloves)
蒼朮	*Ts'ang-shu* (or *Ts'ang-chu*)	Atractylis ovata
草菓	*Ts'au-kuo*	Amomus medium (Ovoid Chinese cardamom)
草蔲頭	*Ts'ao-tou-k'ou*	Amomum costatum
草烏瀉	*Ts'ao-wu-t'ou*	Aconite
澤瀉	*Tse-hsieh*	Alisma plantago
從蓉	*Ts'ung-jung*	Aeginetia Sp.
杜仲	*Tu-chung*	Bark of an Euphorbiaceous tree
土茯苓	*T'u-fu-ling*	Root of the smilax (China-root)
獨活	*Tu-huo*	Angelica inaequalis
兔絲子	*T'u-ssu-tzu*	Cuscuda (Dodder) seeds
芡實	*Tz'u-shih*	Euryale ferox
紫蘇	*Tzu-su*	Perilla ocymoides
威靈仙	*Wei-ling-hsien*	Clematis sp.
五加皮	*Wu-chia-p'i*	Eleutherocrocus
吳茱萸	*Wu-chu-yu*	Evodia rutaecarpa
五靈脂	*Wu-ling-chih*	Magpie's dung
五倍子	*Wu-pei-tzu*	Nut-galls of Rhus semialata
烏藥	*Wu-yao*	Daphnidium myrrha

| 茵陳 | *Yin-ch'en* | Artemisia sp. |
| 遠志 | *Yuan-chih* | Root and root bark of Polygala sibirica |

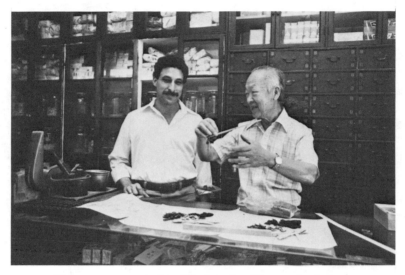

Having a prescription filled at the Chinese herbalist.

Appendix B
TRADITIONAL CHINESE ANATOMY CHARTS

A. The Spleen

B. 1. The lungs have six "leaves" and two "ears," altogether eight leaves.
   2. The Lungs

C. The Pericardium

D. 1. The *Lan* Door (Ileo-caecal valve)
   2. The Large Intestines
   3. The *Kang* Door (Anus)

E. The Heart

F. 1. The *Pen* Door (Cardiac orifice)
   2. The Stomach
   3. The *Yu* Door (Pylorus)

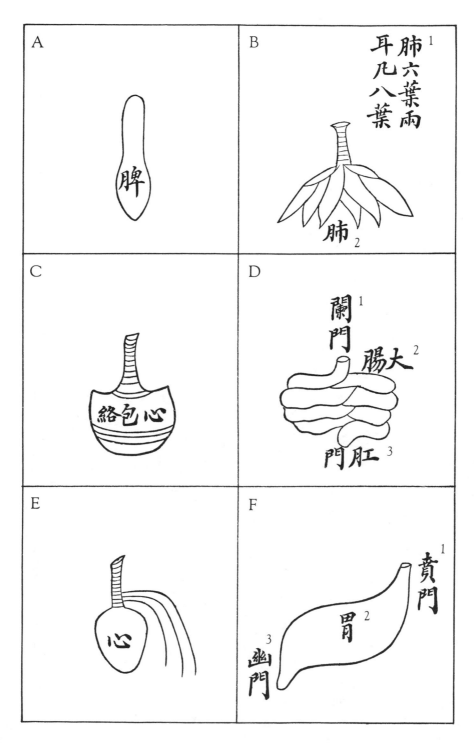

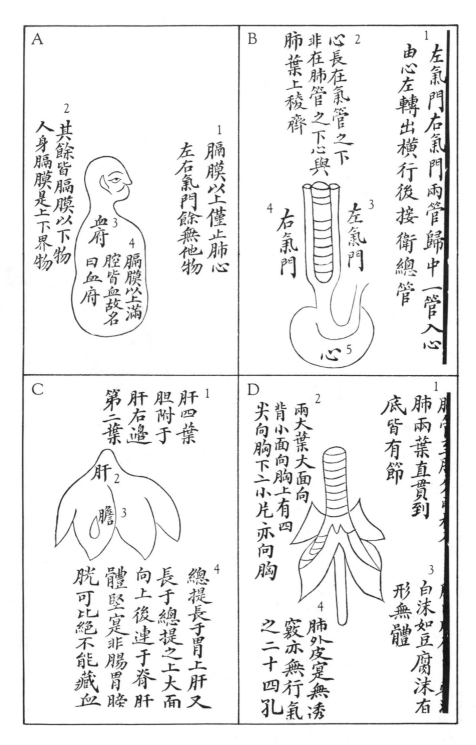

A. 1. Above the diaphragm are only the lungs, heart, and left and right *ch'i-men* ("air doors"); there is nothing else.
   2. All other things are below the diaphragm; in the human body, the diaphragm is the partition between things above and those below.
   3. The *Hsueh-fu* ("blood reservoir")
   4. Above the diaphragm, the chest is filled with blood, and therefore it is called the *hsueh-fu* ("blood reservoir").

B. 1. The two ducts of the left and right *ch'i-men* ("air doors") return to the center and become one duct, which enters the heart. From the left side of the heart, this turns and exits horizontally, connecting behind with the *wei-tsung* duct.
   2. The heart is below the air duct, not below the lung duct (trachea). The edges of the heart are on the same level as the leaves of the lungs above.
   3. The Left *Ch'i-men* ("air door")
   4. The Right *Ch'i-men* ("air door")
   5. The Heart

C. 1. The liver has four leaves. The gall bladder is enclosed in the second leaf on the right side of the liver.
   2. The Liver
   3. The Gall Bladder
   4. The *tsung-t'i* [pancreas?] is above the stomach; the liver is above the *tsung-t'i*. Its large surface is directed upwards; it is connected behind to the spine. The body of the liver is solid; it cannot be compared to the intestines, stomach, and bladder. As a result, it is unable to store blood [as the ancients stated].

D. 1. When the lung duct (trachea) reaches the lungs, it divides into two branches, which enter the lungs' two leaves and go straight down to their bases. [The lung ducts] both have joints (cartilaginous rings).
   2. The large surfaces of the [lungs'] two large leaves are directed toward the back; the small surfaces are directed toward the chest. Above are four points directed toward the chest; below is one small strip which is also directed toward the chest.
   3. What exists within the lungs is a very light white foam like bean curd. The foam has form but no substance.
   4. The outer skin of the lungs is solid and has no openings. Thus there are not twenty-four holes for the passage of air [as the ancients stated].

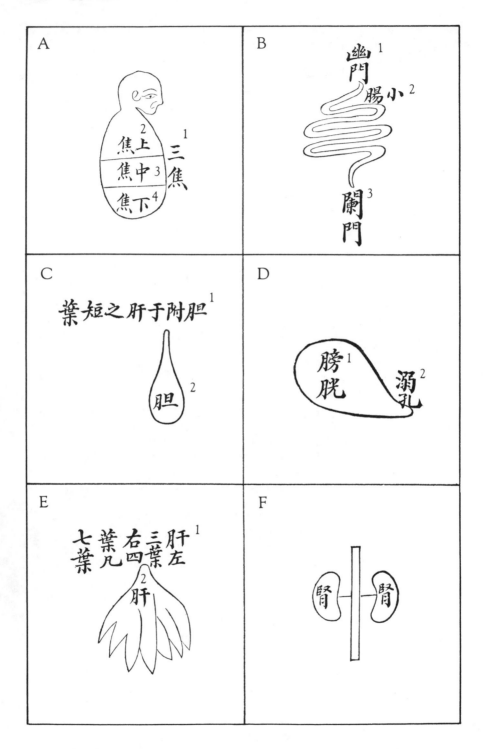

A. 1. The *San Chiao* ("Three Warmers" or "Triple Heaters")
   2. The Upper Warmer
   3. The Middle Warmer
   4. The Lower Warmer

B. 1. The *Yu* Door (Pylorus)
   2. The Small Intestines
   3. The *Lan* Door (Ileo-caecal valve)

C. 1. The gall bladder is enclosed in the short leaf of the liver.
   2. The Gall Bladder

D. 1. The Bladder
   2. The Urethral Canal

E. 1. The liver has three leaves on the left and four leaves on the right, altogether seven leaves.
   2. The Liver

F. The Kidneys

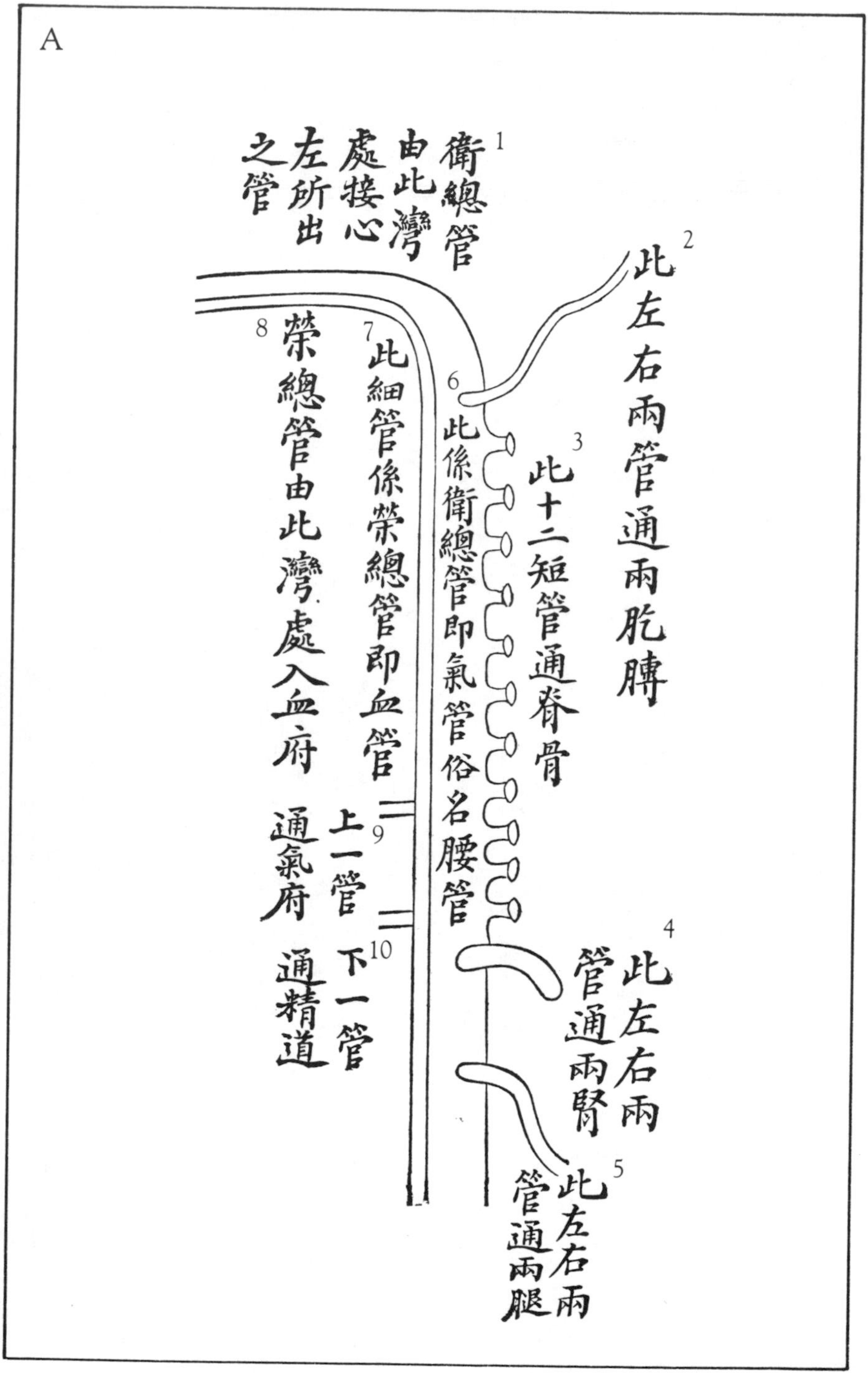

A

1 衛總管由此灣處接心左所出之管

2 此左右兩管通兩肐膊

3 此十二短管通脊骨

4 此左右兩管通兩腎

5 此左右兩管通兩腿

6 此係衛總管即氣管俗名腰管

7 此細管係榮總管即血管

8 榮總管由此灣處入血府

9 上一管 通氣府

10 下一管 通精道

A. 1. The *wei-tsung* duct follows this curve and connects with the duct which exits from the left of the heart.
   2. These two ducts [subclavian arteries], left and right, connect with the two shoulders.
   3. These twelve short ducts [intercostal arteries?] connect with the spine.
   4. These two ducts [renal arteries], left and right, connect with the two kidneys.
   5. These two ducts [iliac arteries], left and right, connect with the two thighs.
   6. This is the *wei-tsung* duct, which is an air duct commonly known as the *yao* [lumbar] duct.
   7. This slender duct is the *jung-tsung* duct, which is a blood duct [vessel].
   8. The *jung-tsung* duct follows this curve and enters the *hsueh-fu* ("blood reservoir").
   9. The upper duct connects with the *ch'i-fu* ("air reservoir").
   10. The lower duct connects with the *ching-tao* ("seminal road").

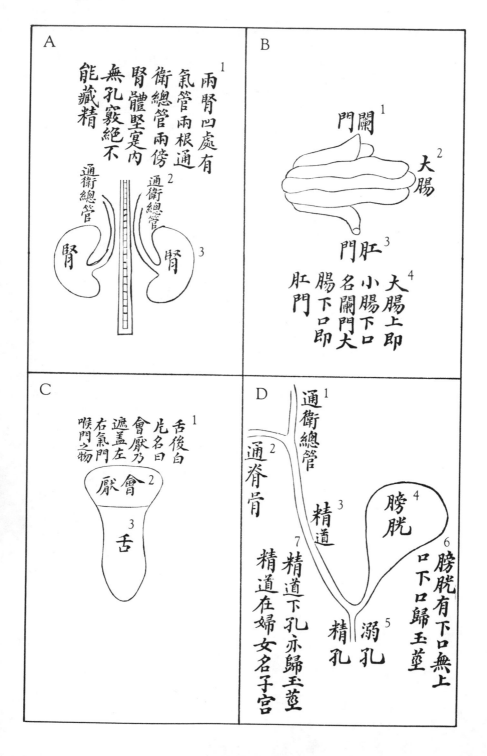

A

兩腎凹處有
氣管兩根通
衛總管兩傍
腎體堅定內
無孔竅絕不
能藏精

1 氣管
2 通衛總管
3 腎

通衛總管
腎

B

1 闌門
2 大腸
3 肛門
4 大腸上即
小腸下口
名闌門大
腸下口即
肛門

C

1 舌後白
片名曰
會厭乃
遮蓋左
右氣門
喉門之物
2 會厭
3 舌

D

1 通衛總管
2 通脊骨
3 精道
4 膀胱
5 溺孔
精孔
6 膀胱有下口無上
口下口歸玉莖
7 精道下孔亦歸玉莖
精道在婦女名子宮

A. 1. In the cavity of the two kidneys are two air ducts which connect with the *wei-tsung* dung. The bodies of the two kidneys are solid; there are no openings within them. As a result, they cannot store semen [as the ancients stated].
   2. Connection to the *wei-tsung* duct
   3. The Kidneys

B. 1. The *Lan* Door (Ileo-caecal valve)
   2. The Large Intestines
   3. The *Kang* Door (Anus)
   4. The upper mouth of the large intestines is the lower mouth of the small intestines; it is called the *lan* door (ileo-caecal valve). The lower mouth of the large intestines is the *kang* door (anus).

C. 1. The white piece at the back of the tongue is called the *hui-yen* (epiglottis). It covers the left and right *ch'i-men* ("air doors") and the *hou* door (larynx).
   2. The Epiglottis
   3. The Tongue

D. 1. Connection to the *wei-tsung* duct
   2. Connection to the spine
   3. The *Ching-tao* ("Seminal road")
   4. The Bladder
   5. The Urethral Canal
   6. The bladder has a lower mouth but no upper mouth. The lower mouth returns to the penis.
   7. The opening at the bottom of the *ching-tao* ("seminal road") also returns to the penis. The *ching-tao* in the female is called the *tzu-kung* (uterus).

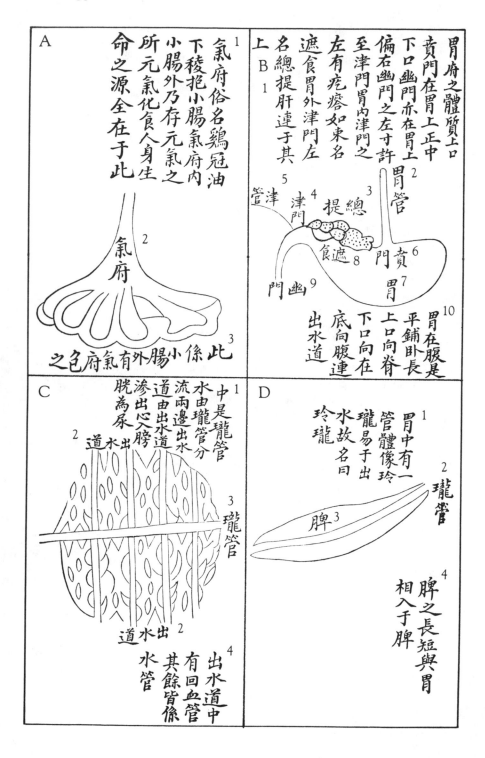

A

氣府俗名雞冠油
下稜把小腸氣府內
小腸外乃存元氣之
所元氣化食人身生
命之源全在于此

氣府

此
係小腸外有氣府包之

B

胃府之體質上口
賁門在胃上正中
下口幽門亦在胃上
偏右幽門之左寸許
至津門胃內津門之
左有疙瘩如柬如
遮食胃外津門左
名總提肝連于其
上

津管　津門　總提　胃管
食遮　賁門　胃　幽門
出水道

胃在腹是
平鋪臥長
上口向脊
下口向在
底向腹連
出水道

C

中是瓏管
水由瓏管分
流兩邊出水
道由出水道
出水
滲出入膀
胱為尿

水出道　瓏管　出水道

出水道中
有回血管
其餘皆像
水管

D

胃中有一
管體像玲
瓏易于出
水故名曰
玲瓏

瓏管
脾

脾之長短與胃
相入于脾

A. 1. The *ch'i-fu* ("air reservoir") is commonly called the *chi-kuan-yen* ("cockscomb oil"). Its lower edge touches the small intestines. Inside the *ch'i-fu* and outside the small intestines is the *yuan-ch'i* ("primordial air"). This *yuan ch'i* digests food; the source of the life of the human body resides entirely here.

2. The *Ch'i-fu* ("Air reservoir")

3. These are the small intestines, which the *ch'i-fu* covers on the outside.

B. 1. The upper mouth of the stomach is the *pen* door (cardiac orifice); it is in the exact center of the upper part of the stomach. The lower mouth, the *yu* door (pylorus), is also in the upper part of the stomach, but on the right side. About an inch to the left of the *yu* door is the *chin* door. Inside the stomach on the left of the *chin* door is a nodule like a bundle called the *che-shih*. Outside the stomach to the left of the *chin* door is called the *tsung-t'i* [pancreas?]. The liver is connected to its upper part.

2. The Esophagus

· 3. The *Tsung-t'i* [Pancreas?]

4. The *Chin* Door

5. The *Chin* Duct

6. The *Pen* Door (Cardiac orifice)

7. The Stomach

8. The *Che-shih*

9. The *Yu* Door (Pylorus)

10. The stomach is spread out flat in the abdomen. Its upper mouth is directed toward the back; its lower mouth is directed toward the right. Its base is directed toward the abdomen and is connected with the *ch'u-shui-tao* ("outgoing water road").

C. 1. In the middle [of the spleen] is the *lung* duct. From the *lung* duct, water divides and flows out on both sides into *ch'u-shui-tao* ("outgoing water roads"). From the *ch'u-shiu-tao*, it percolates out of the heart, enters the bladder, and becomes urine.

2. The *Ch'u-shiu-tao* ("Outgoing water roads")

3. The *Lung* Duct

4. In the middle of the *ch'u-shui-tao* are *hui-hsueh* ("returning blood") ducts; all the rest are water ducts.

D. 1. In the middle of the stomach [spleen?] is a duct shaped like a *ling-lung* [a gem carved with openwork]. This makes it easy for the water to pass out, and thus it is called the *ling-lung* [duct].

2. The *Lung* Duct

3. The Spleen

4. The vessels of the spleen and the stomach enter the spleen together.

Appendix C
ILLUSTRATED EXERCISE TECHNIQUE

Rules To Follow While Practicing:

1. Use common sense when practicing exercises. Do not overexert yourself.
2. Wait three hours after eating before exercising.
3. Work out in a clean, quiet, and well-ventilated environment.
4. Relax your body and free your mind of extraneous thoughts.
5. Do not let your eyes wander while exercising.
6. Breathe naturally through your nose in concert with your movements. Close your mouth lightly and touch your tongue to your palate.
7. Take care of your total health.

STANDING POSTURE FOR MEDITATING

   This on-guard fighting posture can be used to good advantage to strengthen the whole system. Hold each side for 5–15 minutes, changing legs when tired. Add time slowly as strength increases. Breathe naturally and let your body relax. This will become easier with continued practice. As your mind slowly stops thinking, a state of meditation will occur. As you tire, stand slightly higher with your back vertical. You may feel spontaneous movements (or energy) in your body. Do not let these scare you—they will pass in time. If you feel faint or dizzy, stop at once. This standing form is hard work, so proceed slowly.

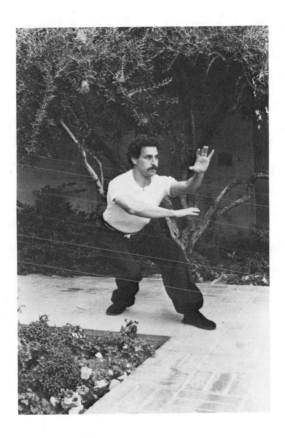

DEEP-BREATHING EXERCISE

Start with arms in front of your body, and with your hands positioned 6 inches in front of your upper thighs (photo 1). Inhale evenly, taking about 7 seconds to fill your lungs completely with air. Simultaneously raise your arms in front of your torso to the fully extended position shown in photo 2. Imme-

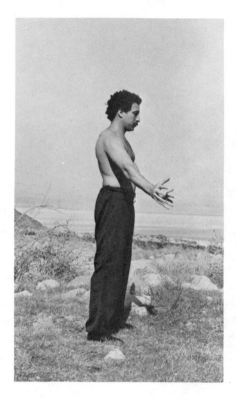 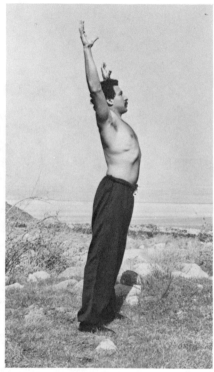

diately start exhaling evenly, taking about 7 seconds to let all the air escape; at the same time lower your arms slowly to the side, ending in the position illustrated in photo 3. Make certain that you force the last bit of air out by pulling in the lower abdomen as you exhale. This is one cycle. Do 10–50 cycles per day, but do not strain.

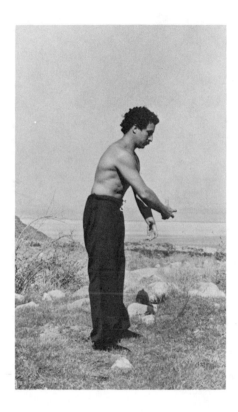

INTERNAL HEALTH EXERCISE

Stand as illustrated in photo 1. Breathe naturally. Inhale slowly while moving the left arm up and the right arm down, and twisting the torso as shown in photo 2. Turn your head to the right until you see your left heel. Stop and hold

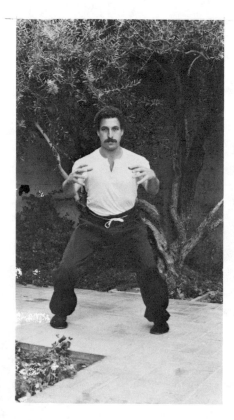
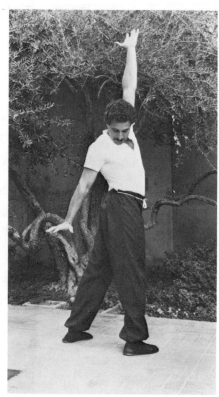

your breath for a few seconds. The finger tips of the high hand point to the front; those of the low hand point to the rear. Both wrists are fully bent. Exhale slowly and return to the position shown in photo 1. Pause for a few seconds. Repeat the exercise, but this time lift the right hand (photo 3). One complete cycle left and right should take about 30 seconds. Continue for several minutes.

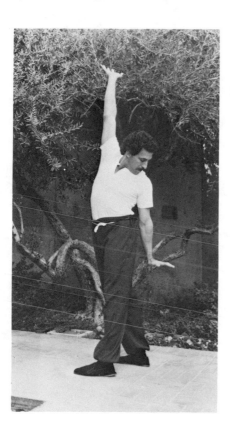

TIGER PLAYING WITH BALL

Turn your body slowly from left to right while exhaling. Your movements should be very fluid. Inhale, reverse your hands, and repeat the motion while moving from the right to left. Your eyes should watch your movement. Continue for several minutes, or until tired.

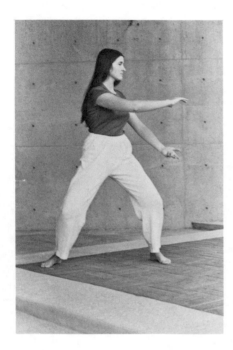 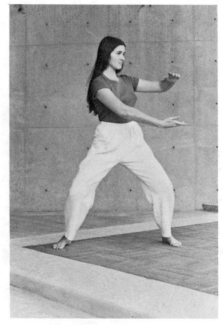

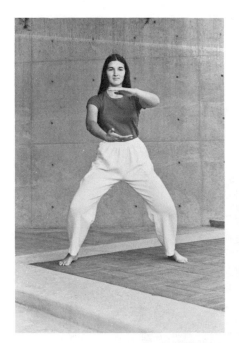
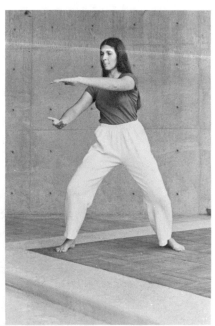
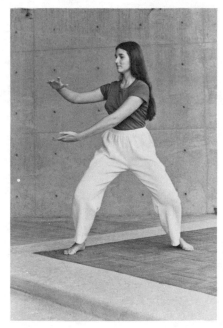

BREATHING EXERCISE FOR WOMEN

This exercise is good for increasing vitality and circulation, menstrual irregularity, and as a post-partum exercise. The best time to do the routine is early in the morning, upon waking.

Inhale slowly as you pull your toes back, taking 7 seconds (photo 1). Exhale slowly while you point your toes, taking 7 seconds (photo 2). During the exercise rub your lower back and kidney area with the backs of your hands, using a small circular motion. Continue for 10–20 minutes, or until tired.

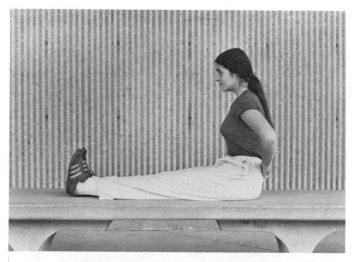

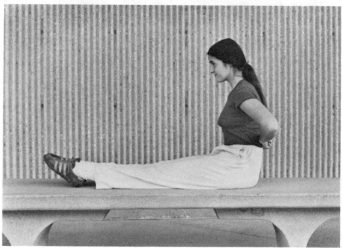

TORSO BEATING

Rotate your waist back and forth while your arms, which are totally relaxed, swing freely. Let your hands and forearms slap your front and back. Breathe naturally. Continue for 1–3 minutes. Be careful not to beat your body too hard at first.

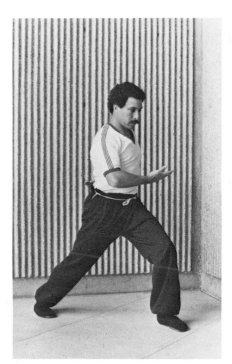 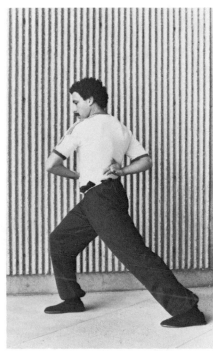

ARM AND LEG TENDON AND MUSCLE BEATING

Walk slowly forward while alternately swinging and beating forearms and instep. After a few months of practice, the exercised parts of your body will become much stronger and resilient. Continue for 1–3 minutes, covering the area from the elbow to the wrist, and from the upper-calf to the lower-calf tendon. Proceed slowly.

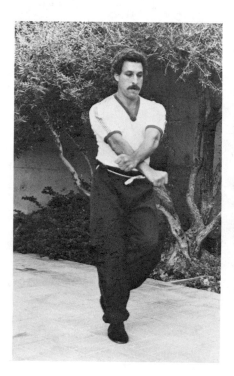 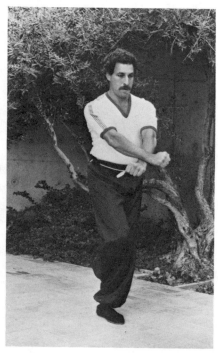

A simple isolation exercise. One of many.

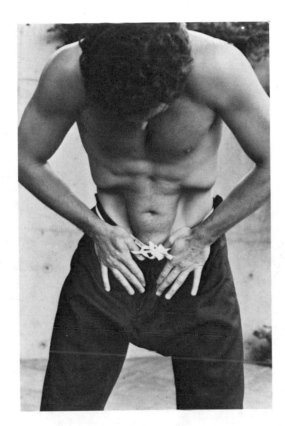

HIP, BACK, AND ABDOMINAL EXERCISES

Exercise A

Position your body as illustrated in photo 1. Rest your palms flat on the ground, under your lower back. Relax, breathing naturally through your nose. Inhale deeply. Let your lower belly expand as you inhale, and remain fully expanded as you hold your breath. Raise your hips to the position shown in photo 2. Hold position for 10 seconds. Exhale slowly as you return to the ground, letting your belly retract in concert with your exhalation. Repeat 5–10 times a day.

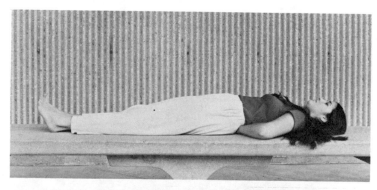

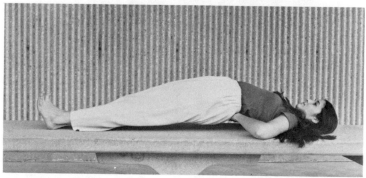

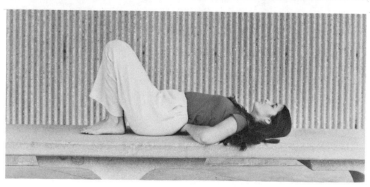

Exercise B

Inhale deeply. Hold your breath as in Exercise A. Raise your hips as in photo 2. Balance on your toes, and hold the position for 10 seconds. Exhale and return to the starting position (photo 1). Repeat 5–10 times.

Exercise C

Inhale as before. Hold your breath; raise your legs and torso to the position shown in photo 2. Hold for 10 seconds. Return to starting position (photo 1). Repeat 5–10 times.

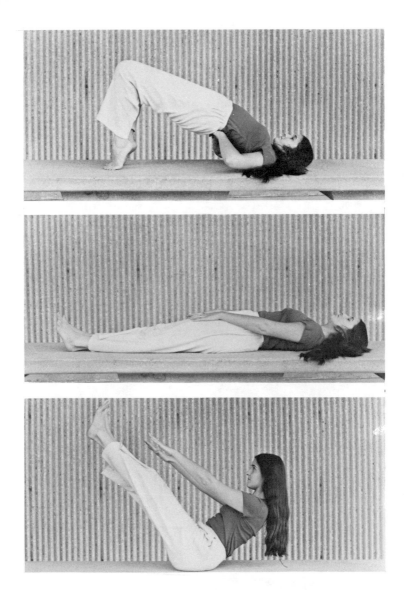

William R. Berk has been practicing martial arts twenty years, and studying Chinese herbal medicine nine years. He has studied with several masters of Chines Internal Kung-Fu and Medical Arts, from both China and the United States. Mr. Berk has studied and taught extensively, including five years at the college level.

UNIQUE LITERARY BOOKS OF THE WORLD

Also publishers of:
Inside Karate
Inside Kung-Fu

UNIQUE PUBLICATIONS
4201 Vanowen Place
Burbank, CA 91505

PLEASE WRITE IN
FOR OUR LATEST CATALOG